*A Remarkable Medicine
Has Been Overlooked*

*When this book was published by Pocket Books
in 1982, quotations from the lay and medical
press were included. They are reprinted here.*

"The Foundation's efforts to examine PHT in such extraordinary detail represents the first time in medical history that a single substance has been so thoroughly investigated as a potential remedy for such a variety of aches and ills."
— Albert Rosenfeld, *Science 81*

" 'Jack Dreyfus, Maverick Wizard Behind the Wall Street Lion' was the title of a long article in Life back in 1966... His book is sure to become a classic."
— Harry Schwartz, *Fortune*

"How Jack Dreyfus became acquainted with this remarkable medication is a story that's exciting and full of human drama. It should be a bestseller."
— *The Berkshire Eagle*

"As a rule, I'm not much for battle stories. But *A Remarkable Medicine Has Been Overlooked* is an exception. Dreyfus deserves our admiration for his truly heroic efforts."
— Ruth B. Schwartz, *The American Council on Science and Health*

(Continued)

"Dreyfus, a winning competitor in whatever he attempts
...The book contains an exhaustive bibliography and
abstracts fom 2,140 published references to PHT research."
—*Medical World News*

"A man who cannot be overlooked...Dreyfus tells the
story of his experiences with simplicity and humor..."
—*MD Magazine*

"I believe this book is a labor of love by a man who has
chosen to take on the established mode of looking at
things that often precludes fresh thinking."
—Susanne Harvey, *Pharmaceutical Executive*

"This successful author is the founder of the Dreyfus
Mutual Fund, a power on Wall Street. How he got out
of his Wall Street business to establish and work in a
charitable medical foundation is a story in itself...a
service to physicians."
—Beth Harris, *Desert Sun*

"This remarkable man has sketched in simple and beautiful prose the story of his life..."
—Ray Kerrison, *New York Post*

"Nobody doubts that Dreyfus has a good deal more than a lick of sense...His message is simple: PHT, best known as the antiepilepsy drug Dilantin, has been shown rigorously to be useful for the treatment of more ailments than any other compound known to medical science."
—William Hines, *Chicago Sun-Times*

"A book with a dramatic and often spellbinding quality —on the side of the angels."
—Peter Schwed, *Turning the Pages*

The Dreyfus Medical Foundation is a
charitable foundation and has no
financial interest in phenytoin.

A
Remarkable
Medicine
Has Been
Overlooked

JACK DREYFUS

DREYFUS MEDICAL FOUNDATION

This book is dedicated to
Mark Twain, to Helen Raudonat,
to Joan Personette, and to Johnny.

Deep appreciation for their friendship and help is expressed to:

DR. J. ANTONIO ALDRETE

DR. WALTER C. ALVAREZ

DR. NATASHA P. BECHTEREVA

DR. LAWRENCE G. BODKIN

DR. SAMUEL BOGOCH

JAMES H. CAVANAUGH

DR. JONATHAN O. COLE

DR. THEODORE COOPER

DR. STUART W. COSGRIFF

DR. JOSE M. R. DELGADO

DR. CHARLES EDWARDS

DR. JOEL ELKES

HON. JOHN W. GARDNER

DR. ELI GOLDENSOHN

DR. PAUL GORDON

DR. LIONEL R. C. HAWARD

DR. RICHARD H. HELFANT

DR. A. D. JONAS

DR. PAUL L. KORNBLITH

DR. HERBERT L. LEY

STUART W. LITTLE

DAVID B. LOVELAND

ALBERT Q. MAISEL

VIVIAN J. McDERMOTT

PROF. RODOLFO PAOLETTI

DR. TRACY J. PUTNAM

DR. OSCAR RESNICK

HON. ELLIOT L. RICHARDSON

HON. NELSON A. ROCKEFELLER

ALBERT ROSENFELD

DR. LAWRENCE C. SCHINE

DR. ALEXANDER M. SCHMIDT

DR. MAXIMILIAN SILBERMANN

HOWARD STEIN

DR. ALFRED STEINER

DR. JOSEPH H. STEPHENS

DR. PETER SUCKLING

DR. WILLIAM H. SWEET

DR. WALTER R. TKACH

DR. WILLIAM J. TURNER

HON. CASPAR W. WEINBERGER

This book was published in 1981 by Simon & Schuster, and by Pocket Books in 1982. Those editions contained Bibliographies and Reviews. The present edition does not, since it was published as a companion piece to *The Broad Range of Clinical Use of Phenytoin*.

With few revisions, this is the same book published in 1981. The story is as pertinent now as it was then.

Prescription medicine

PHT is a prescription medicine, which means it should be obtained through a physician. Nothing in this book should be mistaken to suggest that it be obtained in any other way.

Terminology

The drug that is the subject of this book is known by two generic names, diphenylhydantoin and phenytoin. Phenytoin (PHT) is used in this book.

TO THE READER

Dear Reader:

In 1963 a great piece of luck led me to ask my physician for a medicine that was not supposed to be useful for symptoms I had. It took me out of a miserable condition. When I saw others have similar benefits, I had the responsibility of getting the facts to the medical profession. This was not as easy to do as I thought. I had to leave my businesses in Wall Street. A medical foundation was established. Soon it became apparent that the medicine had been overlooked for a wide variety of disorders.

This book begins with a letter to President Reagan in which this matter is outlined, and his help is sought. The rest of the book is divided into two parts. The first part, a narrative, describes my personal experiences with this medicine. The second part, medical and scientific, contains two bibliographies, *The Broad Range of Use of Phenytoin*, published in 1970, and *PHT, 1975*, prepared by the Dreyfus Medical Foundation and sent to physicians in the United States.*

For eight years, from 1966 through 1973, I did all I could to awaken the Federal government to its obvious responsibilities in this matter—with little success. When the second bibliography had been sent to physicians, it seemed that all a private foundation could do had been

---

* The medical information is not included in this edition since, as has been explained, it was republished to accompany *The Broad Range of Clinical Use of Phenytoin*.

done. And there was progress, but it was slow. Something was wrong.

It's a national pastime to look for culprits. I looked for culprits but I didn't find individual ones. It took me a long time to realize that the culprit was a flaw in our system of bringing prescription medicines to the public.

The only option left was for me to write about my experiences and explain the flaw in our system—for the public, the physician, and health officials, all at the same time. That might get something done.

Nowadays, when you start to read a book, a hand reaches out of the TV set and takes it off your lap. Since this book is about health, you might consider cracking the hand across the knuckles and keep on reading.

Good luck,

JACK DREYFUS

The President
The White House
Washington, D.C.

DEAR MR. PRESIDENT:

I write you about a matter of such urgency and importance that it requires the attention of your office.

The properties of a remarkable and versatile medicine are being overlooked because of a flaw in our system of bringing medicines to the public. This is to the great detriment of the health of the American public, and many millions of people suffer because of it. This tragic condition can be remedied.

This letter is meant as a briefing, Mr. President. Material outlined in it will be expanded on elsewhere.

The medicine is a prescription medicine. Its best known trade name is Dilantin; generic, phenytoin (PHT). The first disorder for which it was found useful was epilepsy. This was in 1938. In those days it was customary to think of a single drug for a single disorder, and PHT promptly got the tag "anticonvulsant."

Since this early discovery, over two thousand medical studies have demonstrated PHT to be one of the most widely useful drugs in our pharmacopoeia. Yet today, forty-one years later, PHT's only listed indication-of-use with the Food and Drug Administration is as an anticonvulsant. This description is accurate but tragically misleading—and plays a major role in the misunderstanding of PHT by the medical profession.

It should be emphasized that this is not the fault of the FDA.

Two lists have been placed in the Appendix (p. 146–50) for your convenience. If you will glance at them now, it will give you an idea of the breadth of use of PHT. One list is comprised of over fifty symptoms and disorders for which PHT has been reported effective.* The other list shows the names of over 250 medical journals, published throughout the world, in which these studies have appeared.

When we see the number of symptoms and disorders for which PHT has been found therapeutic, our credulity is strained. Nothing could be that good, we say. But then we look closer, and we reevaluate. In number the studies are overwhelming. Not having been sponsored by a drug company they were spontaneous and independent, the authors' only motivation being scientific interest and a desire to help others.

A brief discussion of the basic mechanisms of action of phenytoin will be helpful. A general property of PHT is that it corrects inappropriate electrical activity in the body, even at the level of the single cell. When we consider that all our body functions are electrically regulated, our messages of pain are electrically referred, and our thinking

---

* New uses continue to be reported.

processes are electrically conducted, it makes it easy to understand PHT's breadth of use.

Although PHT corrects inappropriate electrical activity, in therapeutic amounts it does not affect normal function. Thus it can calm without sedation and effect a return of energy without artificial stimulation. PHT is not habit-forming, and its parameters of safety have been established over a forty-year period.

You may ask, Mr. President, why I haven't brought this matter to the Department of Health or the Food and Drug Administration. Well, that was the first thing I thought of years ago. And for eight years I spent an eternity with officials in government, being shuffled back and forth from one to another with encouragement and even compliments. During this period I saw three secretaries of HEW, two assistant secretaries of HEW, two commissioners of the FDA, members of the staff of the FDA, a surgeon general, and other officials.

It took me a long time to realize this was the wrong approach. Although everyone agreed that something should be done, no official seemed to think he had the authority or responsibility to get it done. (See Travels with the Government, Chapter 9.)

About the flaw in our system for bringing prescription medicines to the public:

Years ago doctors concocted their own remedies, but that's in the past. Today the origination of new drugs is left to the drug companies—motivated by that reliable incentive, the desire to make profits. Between the public and the drug company is the FDA.

The FDA was set up to do for many individuals what they could not do for themselves. Although its broad purpose was to improve the health of our citizens, it was set up as a defensive agency, to protect against ineffective drugs and those more dangerous than therapeutic, and was not equipped to reach out for an overlooked drug.

Since 1938 drug companies have been required to seek approval from the FDA as to the safety of new drugs and, since 1962, approval of both safety and effectiveness. When an FDA listing is granted it entitles a company to promote a drug for the purposes for which it has been approved. If the drug sells well the company has a good thing. Patent protection gives up to seventeen years of exclusive use. During this period profit margins are high. When patents expire, the financial incentive to look for a new drug is far greater than it is to study new uses of an old drug.

The process patents on PHT expired in 1963—and much of the incentive to do research on the drug expired at the same time. It should be noted that Parke-Davis, the company that had the patents on PHT, did not synthesize the drug and physicians outside the company discovered it to be therapeutic. There is reason to believe that Parke-Davis never understood their own product. In addition to no patent incentive, this could be a reason they have not applied to the FDA for new uses.*

The public's access to a prescription medicine is through the physician. Physicians get their information about prescription medicines from the drug companies, through advertisements and salesmen, and from the *Physicians' Desk Reference,* which carries only those uses for a drug that are listed with the FDA.

---

* One exception, see Chapter 11, p. 112.

One can see how an FDA listing may carry more weight than is intended. In fact some people think of the lack of FDA approval as the equivalent of FDA disapproval. This is clearly wrong. How could the FDA disapprove a use for a drug if it hasn't even had an application for it?

Let's look at the overall picture. Doctors were taught that PHT is an anticonvulsant. The usual sources that the doctors rely on for prescription medicines only indicate that PHT is an anticonvulsant. Is it any wonder that doctors have PHT out of perspective, and that as far as the public is concerned most of the benefits of PHT might as well not exist?

It is apparent that no drug company is going to apply for new uses of PHT. The clock has run down on that probability. Perhaps the FDA does not have a specific means to reach out for this medicine. But since the FDA's broad purpose is to protect the health of the American public, the neglect of a remarkable drug should be in its province, and a means should be found.

A simple solution would be to put the matter in the hands of those qualified—the 450,000 physicians in this country. The FDA could address itself to the basic mechanisms of action of PHT and list it as a substance effective in the stabilization of bioelectrical activity, and refer the physicians to the literature of their colleagues. There are other solutions. The fact is any official nod from the FDA to the physician would let the light from under the bushel, and PHT would find its own level, pragmatically, by its use vis-à-vis other medicines.

Mr. President, this letter is a public one because it is also meant for government officials in health as well as for physicians and the public. The information in this book, for all to see at the same time, should be helpful if you decide to use the influence of your office in this matter. I hope you will. I think you will.

Respectfully,

Jack Dreyfus

Dreyfus Medical Foundation

This letter to President Reagan was in the original book. It has been repeated here because it gives a good outline of the matter. Since writing the letter, I have met with the President and I believe efforts are being made.

CONTENTS

1.
FROM INSIDE
A DEPRESSION

Until I was in my forties, I never really thought about my nerves—a sure symptom of a person with good nerves. I was president of the Dreyfus Fund and a partner in Dreyfus & Co., with responsibilities in research, in sales, and in management. People would ask, "How do you do all the things you do?" "How do you stand the strain?" I hardly understood the question because at the time I felt no strain.

Sometime in my forty-third year I became aware of a change in myself. At partners' meetings, which I'd used to enjoy, I began to notice that my patience was shorter and I was anxious for the meetings to end. Occasionally I felt a trembling inside me that I didn't understand. On weekend trips to the country it had been my habit to read or take a nap in the car. These trips had been relaxing, but they weren't anymore. My mind would become occupied with pessimistic and aggravating thoughts, thoughts I couldn't turn off.

In 1957 I had spent a few trying weeks with a problem in the stock market. It was resolved successfully, but I had been under a good deal of pressure and needed a vacation. I went to Miami and stayed at the Roney Plaza, a nice old-fashioned hotel that I had visited many times before. Usually after a day or two, with the sun and salt water, I would unwind and relax. But this time I didn't relax.

Some premonition made me invite a good friend, Howard Stein, to come down and join me. Howard accepted, and the next day he was at the Roney. Two days later my depression started.

* * *

I awoke at six o'clock in the morning in a state bordering on terror. The early sun was shining, and the birds were singing. In my room at the Roney I was in the safest of surroundings. Yet I was overwhelmed with fear. The fear couldn't have been greater if a tiger had been clawing at the door. I knew there wasn't any tiger, and common sense told me I was safe. But common sense wasn't in charge—fear was. The fear was so great I was afraid to be alone. I called Howard, at that early hour, and asked if he would come to my room. When he got there I told him I knew it didn't make any sense but I was afraid to be alone.

Howard arranged for me to see a doctor, and a few hours later we were in his office. The doctor said, "Miami is the right place for you. Get some sun, go swimming, play a little golf or tennis, and relax." Normally this would have sounded great. But now this advice didn't seem right, and at two o'clock that afternoon I was on a plane back to New York. Although it was a Saturday and I wouldn't see my doctor until Monday, I hoped more familiar surroundings would make me feel better.

I still remember that trip. The plane was half-filled and I had a seat in a row by myself. Even with a dozen or more people in the plane I felt alone, and was afraid. I wanted to ask one of the stewardesses to sit next to me and keep me company, but I didn't because I thought it would be misunderstood. I couldn't tell a stewardess that I was afraid to sit by myself.

My former wife, Joan Personette, one of my closest friends, met me at the plane, and I spent the weekend at her home in Harrison, New York. It was difficult to explain to Joan how frightened I was. My brain was filled with fearful thoughts I couldn't turn off. Saturday night I slept little. Sunday we went out in the cold weather and roasted hot dogs over a fire—something I'd always enjoyed. But this didn't help. The intense fear never left me.

On Monday morning I saw Alfred Steiner, my family physician. He sent me to a neuropsychiatrist, Dr. Maximilian Silbermann. The first question I asked was, "Have I gone crazy?" I'd never had an experience like this— intense fear without apparent cause. And my mood was so pessimistic that the worst seemed plausible. Dr. Silbermann assured me that I was sane but said he thought I was depressed. I remember that he said, "When people are insane, they may think others are a little off, but they rarely question their own sanity."

That first day Dr. Silbermann asked me what I liked to do, what I really enjoyed. I told him that going to the racetrack was something I enjoyed a lot. He said, "Well, why don't you go to the races tomorrow? Don't worry about business." He also suggested that I not be alone and have someone spend the night with me in my apartment.

The next day I intended to go to the races. But I didn't. They had no appeal for me, and even seemed a problem. That day, when I saw him for the second time, Dr. Silbermann diagnosed my condition as an endogenous depression. He explained that endogenous meant "coming from within," and he differentiated it from a reactive depression, one with an outside cause. He assured me that this condition was temporary and that I would come out of the depression. He said he didn't know how long it would take; it could be gradual or it could happen suddenly. Being told this was important to me intellectually, but emotionally I had a hard time believing it.

That was the beginning of a long and close relationship with Dr. Silbermann. For the next few years I was to see him five or six times a week. From the start Dr. Silbermann told me that good sleep was important for my condition and prescribed sleeping medication. With the help of this medicine I slept soundly, and the benefits of sleep carried over. In the morning I was at my best. As the day wore on my mind became busier and busier with worries and fears, and occasional angry thoughts. Frequently around dusk a little depressive cloud would descend upon me; I would tremble and my hands and feet would get cold.

Seeing Dr. Silbermann almost every day was important to me. In his warm office, with his friendliness and willingness to listen, I would unburden my brain of the thoughts that were tormenting me. But intense fear persisted for almost a year. During that period I was afraid to be alone, and I arranged for my housekeeper to spend the night at my apartment.

Of course I had my business responsibilities, and I asked Dr. Silbermann what to do about them. He told me that people misunderstood depressions, and it might be best not to tell anyone about it. He suggested that I leave it vague and say I would be away from the office for a period of time. But this was in conflict with my sense of responsibility, and I didn't feel right about it. Mark Twain advised, "When in doubt, tell the truth." So I told the truth to my partners and asked them to run things without me for a while. Although I was not aware of feeling better, a realistic source of worry was removed.

Dr. Silbermann advised me to try to get out of the house and keep myself occupied, as long as I could do things that were not abrasive to me. I visited museums. One of my main haunts was the Museum of Modern Art and I had many lunches in the cafeteria there. I became friends with the paintings and with the sculptures in the backyard. The attention I gave these pleasing objects was helpful in taking attention off myself. I had similar benefits from the Central Park Zoo where I spent time with the seals, polar bears, and other nice creatures.

I tried to avoid things that would upset me. I found that my mind would magnify the slightest unpleasantness by some large multiple. Newscasts were anathema to me and I couldn't listen to them. If a busload of children overturned in Nevada the news would be dragged fresh and gory to our attention in New York. I quickly learned that the news, with its disaster *du jour*, made things worse. One piece of news I couldn't avoid was the dog in the Sputnik space capsule. I couldn't get it out of my mind, and I suffered with thoughts of that dog for many weeks.

I gave up watching movies on television. There'd be some sad theme or violent incident that would upset me, and the image of it would stick in my head. I had a similar problem with most books. One author I could always read was Mark Twain. I'm sure I missed many of his subtleties but he never dragged me through unpleasantness.

When I'd been in the depression for about six months

Dr. Silbermann asked me if I thought it might make me feel better to be in a hospital. I said I didn't know but I was willing to try it. So he got me a room at the Harkness Pavilion of Presbyterian Hospital. In the room I noticed that the windows were discreetly barred, and I asked the nurse about this. She explained that sometimes deeply depressed persons had to be protected from themselves.

Fortunately I was not classified as deeply depressed. I had outpatient privileges and walked in the neighborhood a few hours each day. It was cold and I would have a bowl of hot soup in a nice little corner restaurant. During the walks I had plenty of time to think. The conversation with the nurse reminded me that Dr. Silbermann had once tactfully brought up the subject of suicide. Now I gave it honest thought and realized I'd never considered it. Not that life seemed that desirable. At that time everyone was talking about the next rocket to the moon, the first to carry men. In my mood I thought chances for success were almost nil. But I remember thinking if a high authority told me it was for the good of the country I might be willing to make the trip.

After three days in the hospital, not feeling better or worse, I returned home. Each day Dr. Silbermann and I talked over my, mostly imagined, problems. Part of me knew that some of the worries were not logical, but the rest of me couldn't feel it. Max cautioned me not to make any major business decisions while I was depressed because my perspective would be out of kilter. This was good advice. The Dreyfus Fund was small at the time, but quite successful, and the only problems it had were the healthy ones connected with growth. Yet on more than one occasion I wished I could give the Fund away.

My apartment was just a few blocks from Dr. Silbermann's office. Often I would leave for my appointment as much as an hour early and kill time by walking. I usually felt cold, and would seek the sunny side of the street. After the appointment, if it was daylight, I would walk in Central Park. I would still try to stay in the sun. As the shadows moved across the park I would walk faster to keep ahead of them.

During these walks I used to think about my condition. I was aware of daily headaches, frequent stomach irregularity, chronic neck pain, and lack of energy. But my dominant symptom was a turned-on mind that never gave me rest and was always occupied with negative thoughts related to anger and fear. And the fear was the worst.

When you have fear in you, you'll find something to be afraid of or to worry about, even if you have to make it up. This happened to me all the time. I'll give two illustrations.

One Sunday, on Madison Avenue, I saw a woman looking at a dress in a small shop. She seemed to be looking at it longingly, as though she wanted it but couldn't afford it. I felt unhappy for her. The dress looked so old-fashioned and unattractive it made me feel even sadder. Now this woman was a complete stranger. For all I knew she might have been able to buy that block of Madison Avenue. But my mood made me decide she couldn't afford the dress. This unhappy picture stuck in my brain and bothered me for days.

Another incident occurred at a cocktail party. One of the guests, a young girl of seventeen, was introduced as the daughter of a famous movie actress. She mentioned that she would have to leave in a little while because she was taking dancing lessons. The girl seemed plain-looking and I felt sad for her. I knew she didn't have a chance to be successful, and was trying to follow in her mother's footsteps because it was the thing to do. When she left, she kissed us all good-bye. She'd even adopted Hollywood ways, and this made me feel even sadder. I worried about this poor girl for many days. It wasn't really necessary—the "poor girl" was Liza Minnelli.

It is almost impossible to convey to a person who has not had a depression what one is like. It's not obvious like a broken arm, or a fever, or a cough; it's beneath the surface. A depressed person suffers a type of anguish which in its own way can be as painful as anything that can happen to a human being. He has varying degrees of fear throughout the day, and a brain that permits him no rest and races with agitated and frightening thoughts. His mood is low, he has little energy, and he can hardly remember what pleasure means. He's in another country, using a different language. When he uses words such as "worry" and "afraid" he may be expressing deep distress. But these words seem mild to the person whose mood is all right.

* * *

The deepest part of my depression lasted for about a year. Then it lessened gradually and there were periods of improvement. These better periods alternated with periods of mild depression for the next few years. "Mild" depression is plenty unpleasant, but I use the term to distinguish it from severe depression.

It began to look as if chronic depressive periods might be with me for life. Then I had an incredible piece of luck.

2.
AN INCREDIBLE
PIECE OF LUCK

Dr. Silbermann and I had numerous discussions about why I was depressed, without reaching any conclusions. There was a theory, proffered by relatives of mine in Boston, that I was neurotic and needed to be psychoanalyzed. Dr. Silbermann didn't agree that psychoanalysis was what I needed, and as a practical matter felt that it would be too arduous while I was depressed.

On my own, as objectively as I could, I considered my relatives' suggestion. I didn't question that I was neurotic. But I didn't see how that could be the answer. Presumably I'd been neurotic before the depression, yet my nerves had been fine.

I began to notice that changes in my mood frequenly occurred without apparent environmental or psychological cause. And the same stimulus didn't always evoke the same response. Sometimes, while driving in the country, I would see a dead woodchuck on the side of the road. The sight would hit me like a blow and I couldn't get it out of my mind. But on other occasions I'd see a dead woodchuck and react in what seemed a normal way. The difference in reactions couldn't be caused by my being neurotic; my childhood from one to five hadn't changed. It seemed plausible that these disparate reactions were due to changes in my body.

I discussed this with Dr. Silbermann, and he was inclined to go along with the idea that there might be something wrong in my body "chemistry." But Max said that he didn't really know, and emphasized that when he said "chemistry," he was using the word in quotes.

* * *

One night, a seemingly insignificant incident started a chain of events that changed my life. A young woman took my hand and massaged my fingers. I was full of tension at the time. As she pressed my fingertips I felt the tension slip away, and I had the feeling that electricity was going out of my body. This didn't make sense to me. I'd never heard of electricity in the body—but the impression was strong. The next day, a Sunday, the impression of electricity was still with me.

It's a misconception, I believe, that we originate ideas. I used to think we did, but I don't anymore. Too often I find my brain does what it wants—it's on automatic pilot most of the time. That was the case this particular Sunday because, without instruction from me, my brain went into its files and came up with three experiences I'd had with electricity. The first went back almost forty years.

One. When I was a little boy I saw a brass plate with a hole in it, in the baseboard. It aroused my curiosity. I stuck my finger in the hole—and my curiosity was satisfied. The electric shock I got, and the sudden, intense fear that came with it, were indelibly impressed on my memory. I remember that after the shock I had a flat, metallic taste in my mouth.

Two. I had gone into a garage with my former wife to get the car. I picked up an old vacuum cleaner, to get it out of the way, and received an electrical jolt. I said to Joan, "This damn thing shocked me."

"It always does that," she said quietly.

At this calm appraisal I exploded. "What do you mean, 'It always does that!' " and I took Joan by the shoulders and shook her. This was so unlike me that I felt my explosion of anger had been caused by the electricity.

Three. On two successive nights I'd had the same frightening dream, or was it a dream? Each of these nights, before going to sleep, I had intense feelings of fear. The "dreams" occurred early in the morning. I felt that I was awake and couldn't open my eyes. I tried to reach for the table light but couldn't move—in the dream I felt I was frozen with electricity.

Each of these experiences with electricity was associated with a symptom of my depression. As I reviewed them, side by side so to speak, they seemed to be related. Numbers one and three made a connection between electricity and fear. Number two connected electricity with anger. And number one also made a connection with the metallic taste in my mouth which I associated with fear.

The logic of these connections was not clear then. But the pieces held together well enough for me to say to myself, When I see Max on Monday I am going to bring up the subject of electricity.

That Monday my appointment with Dr. Silbermann was after dinner, around ten o'clock. I had some "problems" that I wanted to talk out. It wasn't until late in the hour that I brought up the subject of electricity. I said to Max, "You know, I think my problem is electricity, and electricity causes some people to get depressed, others to bump themselves off, and others to go crazy." I said this as though I meant it, but actually I had little conviction.

At that moment my brain jumped back twenty years to a bridge tournament. My partner and I had got the best of two hands, and one of our opponents, a famous player, P. Hal Sims, made some pointed remarks to his partner. I noticed the partner's neck getting red. As we moved to the next table there was a commotion, and I turned and saw the man on the floor, having convulsions. Someone said he was having an epileptic attack. Now, as I thought back to the attack, the convulsions looked like they had been caused by a series of electrical shocks.

I continued with my hypothesis and said, "And some people have an electrical explosion which we call epilepsy." Max said, "It's curious that you mention epilepsy. We know from brain wave tests that the epileptic has a problem with his body electricity." This was the first time I'd heard that there was such a thing as body electricity. Also, connecting the epileptic to an electrical problem was a direct hit. When I'd started the discussion I thought the odds were 10,000-to-1 against me. But now the odds dropped sharply, and they were realistic enough to make the subject worth pursuing.

I knew a girl who'd had an epileptic attack when she was six. She was now fifteen and seemed to be leading a normal and happy life. She had been given a medicine for her epilepsy and I asked Dr. Silbermann what it was. He told me it was Dilantin.

"Well, why don't I try that?" I asked.

I didn't realize then how crucial Max's answer would be for me. He could easily have said no—and that might have been the end of it. But he said, "You can try it if you like. I don't think it will do you any good, but it won't do you any harm."

That night Max gave me a prescription for Dilantin and told me of an all-night drugstore where I could fill it. He suggested that I take 100 mg before going to bed and skip my sleeping pill. He thought the Dilantin might put me to sleep.

I followed instructions. Around midnight I took 100 mg of Dilantin, and no sleeping pill. Apparently I was dependent on the sleeping medication because when I went to bed I promptly fell awake. Before I finally got to sleep, at four in the morning, I thought, this medicine is a flop. Not until years later did it occur to me that I would not have lain quietly in bed for four hours if I'd had my usual fears. I'd have gotten up and taken the sleeping medicine.

I awoke at eight the next morning and, as Dr. Silbermann had instructed me, took another 100 mg of Dilantin. I had missed half a night's sleep. Sleep was so important that when I saw Max that afternoon, I started to tell him the Dilantin didn't work. Max said, "But you look better than you did yesterday." Then I looked at myself and realized that in spite of the loss of sleep I felt much better. We agreed that I should continue the Dilantin.

The following morning, according to routine, I called Dr. Silbermann. I couldn't make an appointment to see him because I was going to be too busy that day. The next day I was too busy again. The third day, when I was going to make the same excuse, I realized that I wasn't too busy. I was ducking the appointment. It was the first time in five years that I didn't feel a need to see Max.

I saw Dr. Silbermann only three more times in his office. My need for psychotherapy was gone, and we just talked as friends. Max told me he had never heard of PHT being used for the purposes I was using it. And he was a close friend of Dr. Houston Merritt, of Putnam and Merritt, who, twenty years earlier, had discovered the first clinical use for Dilantin. So for a while we were waiting for the phenomenon to go away. At least I'm pretty sure Max was. Intellectually I was too. But my feelings told me things were all right.

On my last visit Max gave me a renewable prescription for PHT. I haven't seen him as a patient since. We've stayed the closest of friends, and frequently have dinner together to swap lies and trade psychotherapy.

From the day I took Dilantin my major symptoms of distress disappeared. I noticed fundamental differences. My brain, which had been overactive and filled with negative thoughts, was calmer and functioned as it did before the depression. The headaches, the stomach distress, the neck pain all disappeared. And my patience returned. I enjoyed partners' meetings again and could sit back and observe someone else getting impatient, which was a switch.

Before taking Dilantin I'd been so tired and worn out I just dragged myself around. Although PHT had a calming effect on me, to my surprise it didn't slow me down. On the contrary my energy returned full force. It was as though the energy that had been wasted in my overactive brain was made available for healthier purposes.

I didn't realize it right away, but my good health had returned. I was neither tranquil nor ecstatic. I was just all right. For the first time in my life I realized how good you feel when you feel "all right."

3.
NEW EVIDENCE
AND A BROADENING
PERSPECTIVE

What had happened to me doesn't happen in real life. You just don't ask your doctor to let you try one drug, out of a pharmacopoeia of tens of thousands, and find that it works. But this did happen. And it happened so casually, in such a matter-of-fact way, that the vast improbability of it didn't occur to me at the time.

Being of the human race, I naturally returned to routine. Much of my new energy went back into the Dreyfus Fund and Dreyfus & Co., as though I were trying to make up for lost time. Still, much of my thinking was on PHT and the intriguing puzzle it presented. There were many questions to be answered.

The first question was whether PHT had been the cause of my return to health. My body might have been due for a recovery and a coincidence could have occurred. But this question was soon answered in the affirmative because I was able to observe benefits from PHT an hour after taking it. A second question, about the safety of the medicine, was answered by Dr. Silbermann. He told me it had side effects but they were rarely serious, and it had been tested by time, millions of people having taken it daily for many years. A question that could not be answered right away was whether the benefits of PHT would last. But as months went by, and I continued to feel well, I gained confidence they would last.

The most important question was a broader question. Could PHT help others as it had helped me? It seemed highly improbable. How could important uses for a medicine be overlooked for twenty years? It didn't make sense, it seemed almost impossible. But if it were so, I clearly had an obligation to do something about it. I needed more facts.

In the course of the next year I was to get more facts. During this period I saw six people, in succession, benefit from PHT. I wasn't looking for these cases. They just happened in front of my eyes, so to speak. Each of the six cases was impressive. But the first two, because they were the first two, had the most significance and will be described in some detail.

*   *   *

The first person I saw benefit from Dilantin was my housekeeper Kathleen Fenyvessy. A month after I had started taking PHT I noticed that Kathleen was not her usual self and seemed depressed. Normally she was energetic but now she seemed worn out. Kathleen, who had recently come from Hungary, spoke imperfect English, and I was in the habit of talking slowly to her. Now she would interrupt before I could finish a sentence, saying, "I understand, I understand"—and most of the time she didn't. Obviously she was extremely impatient.

I asked her what was wrong. She told me her mind was busy with miserable thoughts and she couldn't stop them. She'd seen several physicians and they'd told her she was having a nervous breakdown. She'd tried a variety of medicines that hadn't helped. I thought of PHT. There seemed

little to be lost, and much to be gained, by her trying it—
if Dr. Silbermann agreed. At my suggestion Kathleen visited him. After considering her condition he prescribed
100 mg a day for her.

Since I saw Kathleen at least a few hours every day, I
was in a good position to observe the effects of PHT.
Within a day or two it was apparent that her good disposi-
tion had returned. And she was full of energy again. As for
patience, she no longer interrupted me in mid-sentence. I
could even tell her the same thing twice.

Kathleen found her recovery hard to believe. In a letter to her sister describing it, she said, "It was due to a
medicine used for an entirely different disorder. If someone else had told me they'd had an experience like this I
would not have believed it."

About a month after Kathleen had started taking PHT,
she and I participated in an unplanned experiment. Without consulting each other, we both stopped taking PHT for
three days. We had gone to Hobeau Farm in Ocala, Florida, a thoroughbred breeding farm managed by Elmer
Heubeck, my good friend and partner in the farm. It was
pure vacation for Kathleen. Except for the horse business
it was vacation for me too.

At that time I thought Dilantin only helped me with
stress and problems. By problems I really meant areas of
interest. They were not always problems; when they went
well they could be pleasures. But the negative mood that
I had been in made me think of them as problems. I had
five such interests, some of a business nature, some personal. I went over them; they were all in good shape. So it
seemed to me that in the nice relaxed atmosphere of the
farm, I wouldn't need PHT. I stopped taking it.

The third day off PHT I felt a certain tingling in my

nerves. I remember a funny expression entering my mind, that I had "worry gnats." I thought maybe I'd feel better if I went to Miami, played some tennis and swam in the salt water. So I made arrangements to take a plane to Miami at eleven o'clock that night.

That afternoon I said something to Kathleen. It might not have been as tactful as it should have been, but it couldn't possibly have called for the response that it got. Kathleen burst out crying. I was astonished. Then something occurred to me, and I asked, "Kathleen, have you stopped taking PHT?" She said she had; she'd thought it would be so nice on the farm she didn't bring any. "Why didn't you take some of mine?" I asked. She said she hadn't because she'd noticed I had only a few capsules left. Before I left for Miami, Elmer told me he would arrange for Kathleen to get PHT.

At 11 P.M. I got on the plane to Miami. Now I was quite conscious of the "worry gnats," and I thought of PHT. I figured it wouldn't help since I didn't have any stress or problems. But something inside me said, Well, you're research-minded. Why don't you take some anyway and see if anything happens. My bags were accessible on the plane and I went forward and got a capsule of Dilantin. I took it and looked at my watch. In a little while I thought I felt better, but I wasn't sure. I checked the time; it was twenty-eight minutes since I'd taken the medicine. When the plane arrived in Miami it was an hour since I'd taken the Dilantin. The "worry gnats" were gone. As I walked through the airport I had the nicest feeling that peace had descended on me.

The next morning I called Kathleen. Even before I could ask how she felt, her cheerful voice gave the answer.

Kathleen's experience and my own, in stopping PHT and recontinuing it, confirmed our need for the medicine, and seemed to indicate this need was not based on realistic problems, but on something in our nervous systems at the time.

Now I was in Miami again. I had gone there for the last few years on doctor's orders. These trips were meant to be vacations, but there had been no fun in them. When a vacation is not in you, you don't have one. But now I was on vacation and in a frame of mind to enjoy it. I still stayed at the lovely, dilapidated old Roney Plaza. Everything was beautiful—the air, the sea, just walking to breakfast. I was happy. And I know why. As Mark Twain said in "Captain Stormfield's Visit to Heaven," "Happiness ain't a thing in itself—it's only a *contrast* with something that ain't pleasant." I had the contrast.

Tennis was a pleasure again. I had taken up tennis about eight years earlier, mostly for the exercise. Golf had been my game since childhood and I'd loved it. I'd been almost a fine golfer, won lots of club championships, and at my best had a one handicap. But in recent years golf had started to bore me. Maybe it was my perfectionism. More likely it was the long walks between shots when all that was going on was the windmills of my mind.

I had started playing tennis with the local pros at the Roney Plaza. At this time Marse Fink was pro of record. Sol Goldman was pro emeritus. I didn't play with the pros to get lessons. I'd had barrels of lessons in golf and I looked forward to doing everything wrong in tennis.

We got up all sorts of games and bet on them all. They gave me large handicaps. Sometimes Marse and Sol played doubles against me and some bum they got as my partner.

Sol and Marse were good friends, but if the match got close, they were not loath to comment on each other's play. They called each other names their mothers hadn't taught them. I'd get so interested in their descriptions of each other that I would lose my concentration—and they'd usually win. On the rare occasions they lost, Marse would go to his desk in the tennis shop and mutter to himself, so we could all hear, "I'll never play with that son-of-a-bitch [Sol] again." And he never did—until three o'clock the next afternoon.

Sol and Marse never beat me badly—just consistently. One day they paid me a fine tribute. They told me I was ranked third on the International Sucker List (behind a Frenchman in Monte Carlo and a Greek in Philadelphia). I didn't let this go to my head.

Sol, a remarkable character (the world's leading authority on everything), was the second person I saw benefit from PHT. In his youth Sol was a great athlete, acknowledged to be the best one-wall handball player in the world. When he was thirty he took up tennis and became an outstanding player. In a different field, Sol had ambitions to be an opera singer. He had a fine singing voice and might have made it to the Met if he hadn't damaged a vocal cord.

One morning Sol and I had breakfast at Wolfie's on Collins Avenue. The waitress brought mushroom omelettes and Sol ignored his. He seemed in a fog and was staring into the distance. I'd heard that you could pass your hand in front of someone's face and they wouldn't notice, but I'd never believed this. I passed my hand a few inches in front of Sol's face and didn't get any reaction at all.

I asked Sol what was bothering him. He said that a couple of weeks ago a wealthy friend of his, whom I knew well, had bought six pairs of tennis shoes from Marse. Sol thought it terrible that Marse had charged his friend retail prices for the shoes. This was of such monumental inconsequence that I had a hard time believing the thought was stuck in Sol's brain. But after listening to him I realized that it was almost an obsession. Then it occurred to me that Sol's tennis game had been off, and he'd been uncharacteristically quiet on the court.

I asked Sol how he'd been feeling. He told me he had constant headaches, that he slept badly and was having nightmares. His worst complaint was that he would wake up at four o'clock in the morning hearing himself shouting. His only relief was to get in his car and drive around for an hour or so. He told me he'd seen a doctor. But the medicines he'd been given hadn't helped and made him feel dopey. It seemed that PHT might be worth trying. I telephoned Dr. Silbermann about it, and he arranged for Sol to get a prescription.

The next day we were at Wolfie's again. Sol had eaten earlier and was keeping me company at breakfast. He had his Dilantin with him and took the first 100 mg at that time. I had found PHT effective in myself within an hour, and this was a chance to observe its effects in someone else. I wanted an objective reading but didn't know how to go about it. By chance I asked Sol, "What about Fink and Russell this afternoon?" We had a doubles game with them for fifty dollars a team. Sol said, "They're awful tough." This answer startled me—it was so unlike Sol, a fierce competitor. I thought, "Fink and Russell" will be a good test question. I looked at my watch.

We left Wolfie's and walked to the beach at the Roney Plaza, a couple of blocks away, and I went in swimming.

When I came back it was thirty-five minutes since Sol had taken his PHT. I said, "Sol, do you think we've got a chance with Fink and Russell this afternoon?" Sol said, "We've *always* got a chance." With emphasis on the always. That was more like him.

Twenty-five minutes later, an hour after Sol had taken the PHT, I asked again, "What about Fink and Russell?" Sol said, "We'll knock the crap out of them." Sol was back to normal.

That night Sol slept soundly and straight through. He started taking Dilantin daily and continued to sleep well —no more waking up at four in the morning. His daily headaches disappeared. The monumental matter of the retail shoes shrunk back to size. And once again Sol became his usual objectionable self on the tennis court.

* * *

In that first year I saw four more people benefit from PHT. Each was depressed and each had symptoms of an overbusy brain occupied with emotions related to fear and anger. Because the cases were so important to me summaries of them are included in the Appendix (p. 151).

Each additional one of these cases had a parlaying effect on the probability factor. A year earlier it had seemed almost impossible that important uses for PHT could have been overlooked. Now it seemed highly probable that they had been overlooked.

Which brings up the subject of probabilities.

4.
THE SUBJECT
OF PROBABILITIES

As I look back, I realize that it was a good instinct for probabilities that pulled me through that early period of my pursuit of PHT. Without this instinct I could never have survived the negative inferences drawn from the fact that the medicine had been around for over twenty years. I used to think that everyone had a pretty good sense of probabilities. But I don't now, and I've heard some strange comments about probabilities in the medical field.

Probabilities are an important underlying theme of this book and, partly to qualify myself on the subject, I will depart from the narrative and discuss them.

In some fields a sense of probabilities is much more important than in others. An insurance actuary would feel naked without a sense of probabilities. A painter, on the other hand, might swap his sense of probabilities for a two-percent improvement in color sense. In medicine a sense of probabilities is more important than generally realized. Sometimes weighing the probabilities—the use of a potentially dangerous procedure against the dangerous condition a patient is in—is the whole medical question. In the FDA the weighing of risk vs. gain looms large in the question of whether a drug should be approved for listing.

I've always had a good sense of probabilities—born

with it I believe—and I used to think of it as a form of intelligence. But as I began to assess some of my other "forms of intelligence" and found them lacking, I decided I'd better think of them all as aptitudes.

The word aptitude itself suggests wide variances. It seems that aptitudes come with the baby. We're not all born with a good sense of direction, and a good sense of probabilities is not standard equipment either. On the way to the subject of probabilities, let's discuss aptitudes. If the reader doesn't have a good sense of probability this should make him feel better.

Some of the genetic blanks I drew when aptitudes were being handed out were in mechanics, in remembering names, and in sense of direction.

Things mechanical are a mystery to me. In World War II, I took an exam to qualify for Officers Training School in the U.S. Coast Guard. My aptitude for mechanics helped me get a grade of 29 out of a possible 100. After looking at this score the Coast Guard decided it had enough officers, and awarded me the post of apprentice seaman.

I can't remember people's names no matter how hard I try. I seem to have a scrambling device in my head. If two strangers come into the office, my secretary discreetly writes their names on the side of a paper coffee cup—and I have to refer to it constantly.

My most conspicuous aptitude—in absentia—is my sense of direction. For that reason, and because there is evidence of genetic origin, I will discuss it more fully.

My sense of direction is fine—but it's in backwards. This is not easy to explain to a person with a good sense of direction. I believe such a person has a tug he's not conscious of that pulls him in the right direction. I have such a tug, but it pulls me in the wrong direction. For example, when I leave a washroom in a strange airport, without hesitation I turn the wrong way.

Apparently my aptitude for going the wrong way is not only lateral but vertical. For fifteen years my office was on the twenty-ninth floor of 2 Broadway and our boardroom was on the thirtieth. When I was in a hurry to get to the thirtieth floor I would invariably walk down to the twenty-eighth.

I don't have to climb the family tree very high to see where I got my sense of direction. It was bequeathed me by my father. His sense of direction was in backwards too —and was even stronger than mine. He got lost all the time but it never occurred to him to blame his sense of direction, he just thought it was bad luck. It's a good thing Dad didn't have to make his living as a wagon scout in the old days. He'd have set out for California with his train of covered wagons and, if things went well, in a few months he'd have discovered Plymouth Rock.

It's not surprising that the family hero is the homing pigeon. You can put this rascal in a dark bag, take him 500 miles from home, and without consulting a road map or following the railroad tracks he will fly directly to his coop. Scientists may say he takes radar soundings or something. But what of it? Could Shakespeare do it, could Beethoven? The pigeon has quite an aptitude.

Without realizing it, we gravitate in the direction of our aptitudes. We bounce from one field to another, being repelled or attracted, and if we're lucky we come to rest where our aptitudes are at a premium. When I got out of college, I bounced around for a few years and wound up as assistant to a customer's broker in the stock exchange. The stock market appealed to my sense of probabilities and another aptitude, gambling (speculation as it's called in the market).

An aptitude for gambling by itself is a dubious asset; it's fortunate for me that this aptitude came in a package with my sense of probability. This steered me into games of skill and away from casino games, such as dice and roulette, where the odds against you are slight but inexorable.

My first gambling game was marbles for keeps. I remember bankrupting a kid from down the block when I was six. When I gave up marbles, I took up other games— contract bridge, gin rummy, and handicapping the races. In these games a good sense of probabilities is an asset.

There are two kinds of probabilities. There is the mathematical kind that can be arrived at precisely. As a simple example, the chance of calling the toss of a coin correctly (provided it's not weighted) is exactly one in two. The chance of calling it correctly twice in a row is one-half of one-half of a chance, or one in four, and so forth. If you wish to determine the exact probability that a coin tossed a hundred times will come up heads thirty-one times, there's a formula for it. I don't know it.

Another kind of probability cannot be arrived at by mathematical formula. It's an estimate—exact figures can't be placed on it. Let's call it free-form probability. We use it all the time, some of us more consciously than others. For example, when I make a phone call I start to assess the probability that the person I'm calling is at home. With adjustments for the individual, I might figure it's three-to-one against his or her being home after the third ring, eight-to-one after the fourth ring, etc. After the fifth ring I usually hang up. (When I call my former wife, if the phone is answered before the fourth ring, I know I've got the wrong number.)

One who makes a living by the application of free-form probabilities is the racetrack handicapper. After studying the many variables, he comes up with the probable odds for each horse in a particular race—the morning line. Over a period of time the handicapper's "line" should be close to the odds made by the betting public, or as my friend Dingy Weiss says, "He can tell his story walking."

Free-form probability also deals with odds of a larger magnitude. Some examples. The odds against five horses, in a ten-horse race, finishing in a dead heat. The odds against finding a lion in your backyard in Manhattan. The odds against the next person you meet having a red beard and a wooden leg, and offering you a banana. Or, for a pertinent example, the odds against thousands of physicians, working independently, finding a drug useful for over fifty symptoms and disorders, and that drug being useful for only a single disorder.

When the odds are this large, it's easy to be approximately right. Whether you estimate one chance in a million or one chance in a billion, the estimates are almost the same—the difference between these figures is less than one in a million. (If the reader's sense of probability is like my sense of direction, his feelers will tell him this is wrong.)

High authorities have no problem with this concept. Recently at the Cavendish Club, I found Phil and the Little Beast, top-notch bridge players who bet on anything that moves, discussing a bridge hand. I made myself heard over a cacophony of "hearts," "Ira," and "idiots," and said

I wanted to ask a serious question. "What's the difference between a million-to-one shot and a billion-to-one shot?" The answers shot back. From Phil, "Nuthin'." From the Little Beast, "Darn little—less than one in a million." I thanked them, and joined the bridge discussion.

A feel for probabilities is essential in two of the card games I've played, bridge and gin runny. Although I haven't played gin in fifteen years, the *Encyclopedia of Bridge* is still kind enough to say, "Dreyfus . . . is reputed to be the best American player of gin rummy." This compliment, no longer deserved, is based on a system of play I discovered many years ago that relies heavily on probabilities.

Gin rummy deals mostly with exact probabilities. Another game I've played, the stock market, deals largely with inexact probabilities.

* * *

October. This is one of the peculiarly dangerous months to speculate in stocks in. The others are July, January, September, April, November, May, March, June, December, August, and February.
—Mark Twain, *Pudd'nhead Wilson*

With this cautionary note the reader will be given instructions on how to buy a stock.

Take the five-year earnings record of a company, its current earnings and your estimate for the near future, its book value, its net quick assets, the prospect for new products, the competitive position of the company in its own industry, the merits of the industry relative to other industries, your opinion of management, your opinion of the stock market as a whole, and the chart position of the individual stock. Put all this where you think your brains are, circulate it through your sense of probabilities, and arrive at your conclusion. Be prepared to take a quick loss; your conclusion may be wrong even though you approached it the right way.

My introduction to Wall Street was in 1941. I got a job as an assistant to a customer's broker in the garment district branch of Cohen, Simondson & Company, at a salary of $25 a week. One of my duties in this job was the posting of hundreds of weekly charts. This early experience with charts influenced my Wall Street career.

Skipping the intervening travail—fascinating as it would be to nobody—I found myself, in the early fifties, responsible for the management of a small mutual fund, The Dreyfus Fund. The fund was so small that the management fees were only $3,000 a year. Perforce, the fund could not afford a large research staff. Actually our staff consisted of a fine young man, Alex Rudnicki, and myself. Alex was a fundamentalist, a student of the Graham Dodd school. I was a student of charts and market technique. We were at the opposite extremes of investment approach, but we worked together as friends.

Alex had a wonderful memory for the earnings of companies and other statistical information; my contribution was 600 large-scale, weekly line charts. From my experience, monthly charts were too "slow" to be of much use, and daily charts were too volatile to be reliable. I split the difference with weekly charts, posted daily. I developed my own theories about the charts, and read no books on the subject. It seemed best to make my own mistakes—at least then I'd know who to blame.

In those early days, our statistical information was no more up-to-date than the latest quarterly reports. Alex and I were too chicken to call a company and ask a vice-president how things were going. Of necessity we put more emphasis on the technical side of the market than did most funds.

When you study the technical side of the stock market you deal with two components. One component is major market trends—bull or bear market. The other is the timing of the purchase or sale of individual securities.

In those days, more than now, the market tended to move as a whole—being right about the major trend was more than half the game. We focused a good deal of our attention on this. With three- and four-million-share days, the trading of the speculator was a key factor in market moves. Speculators tended to move in concert. Excessive optimism, with the parlayed purchasing power of their margin accounts, caused the market to get out of hand on the upside; forced selling in these same margin accounts caused the market to get out of hand on the downside.

The more money a speculator had, the healthier the technical side of the market—he had purchasing power. The more stock the speculator had, the weaker the technical side—he had selling power. Human nature being what it is, when a speculator owned stock he talked bullish. When he had cash, or was short of stock, he talked bearish. In estimating whether we were in a major uptrend or downtrend the speculator's chatter was taken into consideration, along with changes in the short interest and the condition of the margin accounts. And of course our charts were helpful.

Objectivity—difficult to come by—is important in any

field. It didn't take us long to learn that stubbornness, ego, and wishful thinking could mess up the best of market techniques; so we tried to keep our emotions separate from our decision-making. When we bought a security we didn't pound the table to emphasize how sure we were that we were right. Instead, we tried to prepare ourselves for the possibility that we might be wrong so that when the unexpected happened, which it usually did, we were psychologically in a position to take a loss.

Our sense of probabilities was always in play. We wouldn't buy a high-risk stock, one that could go down fifty to sixty percent, unless we felt we had a chance of at least doubling our money. If we bought a conservative stock, one not likely to go down more than twenty percent, a thirty percent profit was worth shooting for.

Since our methods differed from those of most other funds, it was likely that our performance would vary considerably from the average. Fortunately for our stockholders this variance was in the right direction—it could have been the other way. At the time of my retirement, our ten-year performance was the best of any mutual fund—nearly 100 percentage points better than the second-best fund.*

That was a long time ago. Recently, my good friend Bill Rogers, of two-Cabinet-post renown, said, "Jack, I guess you're doing well in the market as usual." I said, "No, Bill, to tell you the truth I've been in a long stupid streak." It's nice to see a friend have a good laugh.

* * *

Back to medical probabilities. Including my own case, I had seen seven consecutive persons benefit from PHT.

* 326% to 232%, Arthur Wiesenberger, Inc.

If each case had been the flip of a coin, 50-50, the odds against seven in a row would have been 127-to-1. But the response to PHT had been so prompt and the symptoms that responded so similar, each case deserved a weight far exceeding 50-50.

Of course my objectivity could be questioned. But that didn't bother me; it's only other people's objectivity that bothers me. Even at that early date I placed a high probability figure on the chance that PHT was more than an anticonvulsant.

*   *   *

During the first year of my experience with Dilantin I had gathered some helpful information on the subject of electricity in the body. This will be discussed in the next chapter.

5.
BODY ELECTRICITY

For the first few months that I took PHT I gave little thought to how the medicine worked. How it worked was a lot less important to me than that it did work. But one day I noticed that the flat, metallic taste in my mouth, which I'd associated with electricity, was gone. As I thought back about it, I realized that it had been gone since I'd started taking PHT.

A hypothesis about electricity had led me to ask for PHT. Was this a coincidence? It seemed unlikely. When a hypothesis precedes and leads to a finding, the hypothesis is apt to be correct. My thinking went back to electricity in the body.

Recently I found some notes to myself, made in 1963. These notes help me remember what my thoughts were at that time.

[From my notes:] "I noticed figures of speech that described human emotions in electrical terms. Before then I'd thought of these terms as imaginative inventions of writers. But perhaps they weren't. Maybe sensitive people had used them instinctively because they were near the truth. There are enough of these electrical expressions to make a parlor game. Here are some:

state of tension	shocking experience
room charged with tension	state of shock
get a charge out of something	it gave me a jolt
electrifying experience	blow your fuse
the touchdown electrified	blow your top
the crowd	sparks flew
dynamic personality	explosive temper
magnetic personality	explode with anger
galvanized into action	

"This list, with its references to anger and fear, led to other thoughts. I knew that an electric goad was used in rodeos to frighten animals into rambunctious performances, and that batteries had been used to make race horses run faster. I'd read that an electric jolt causes the hair to stand on end.

"Could electricity be the mechanism that makes the fur on a dog rise when he is angry or when he is frightened? Could it account for the spectacular bristling of a cat in the act of welcoming a dog? How about our own fur? When we're scared the hair on the nape of our neck rises and we have 'hair-raising' experiences. And don't we bristle with anger? Didn't these things seem to connect anger and fear with electricity in the body?" [End of the notes.]

I had gone as far as I could as an amateur. I needed a professional to tell me whether my ideas about electricity in the body made sense. But where could I find such a person?

Whenever I'm stumped as to how to find someone or locate something, I have a simple method. I ask Howard Stein. I don't know how he does it but he never lets me down. I asked Howard, "Do you know how I can meet with somebody who's an expert on electricity in the body?" Howard said he thought so. He went to Yura Arkus-Duntov, head of the Dreyfus Fund's science research. Within a week Yura had made arrangements for me to meet with Dr. Peter Suckling, a neurobiophysicist from Downstate Medical Center.

Dr. Suckling, with his nice Australian accent, had good vibes for me (a modern electrical term?). He was an expert on bioelectrical activity and had been an associate of Sir John Eccles, an authority in the field and a Nobel prize winner.

Dr. Suckling and I had three long meetings in my office at 2 Broadway. It was a nice office, facing New York harbor, and Peter liked it. He said he thought the moving scenery of boats helped with thinking. I hoped so.

The first question I asked Peter was, "Can you weigh the electricity in a cat?" I thought cats had an extra share of electricity, because of their hair-raising act. Peter disappointed me by saying electricity can't be measured that way. It's inside the body, but the whole animal itself is grounded. I didn't know what that meant but I took his word for it.

For the first time, I heard about the excitatory nervous system, the inhibitory nervous system, membranes, axons, synapses, negative potentials, sodium and potassium, and how a disproportionate amount of chemicals inside and outside the cell made for the electrical potential across the membrane.

Peter labored hard to explain the working of bioelectrical activity to me. By using simple illustrations, he got into me, shoehorn fashion, a rudimentary idea of how electricity works in the body. I won't burden the reader with the whole discussion, but I will summarize some of what Peter said.

The cell is a complicated entity in which thousands of activities take place. Peter said most of them were not relevant to our discussion. What was relevant was the electrical potential of the cell. He explained that the body of a cell is enclosed by a membrane, and in a nerve cell the electrical potential is minus 90 millivolts, relative to the outside of the cell. Peter said the reason there is this negative potential is because of a disproportionate amount of substances inside the cell relative to outside the cell—particularly sodium and potassium. Peter spoke of the membrane with obvious admiration: "This very thin membrane can sustain an electrical tension better than most insulators. The insulation strength is high. It has to be strong; it's so very thin." Then, in considerable detail, he explained the electrochemical mechanisms involved in the discharge of electrical activity. I won't go into that here.

Peter said that there are about 10 billion* cells in the brain—each with an electrical potential. He said that even a slight imbalance in individual cells, because of the proliferative possibilities, could cause a problem in a large area of the brain. He told me that cells vary in length in the human. In nerve cells the speed of impulse transmission varies from one hundred meters a second to three meters a second.

All the cells in the human body, although they do not have the same amount of electrical potential, work on the same principle. Peter said this was true in other animals

* This figure was imprecise. The latest census has it considerably higher.

and, for that matter, all living things. Apparently when the Lord came up with a good thing like the cell he used it over and over again.

At the beginning I didn't tell Peter what my interest was. I didn't want to influence him one way or the other. I realized later that this had been a needless precaution because we were dealing with a pretty exact science. In the meantime, Peter had been trying to figure out why the president of a mutual fund and partner of a brokerage firm was asking all these questions. He'd assumed my interest was in business. On the third day, when I told him about PHT, Peter astonished me by saying, "Oh, my goodness, I thought you were considering giving testosterone to the customer's brokers to make them produce better." Perhaps like making hens lay eggs faster (Merrill Lynch—consider).

Then I explained to Peter what my experiences with PHT had been. Apologizing for the unscientific sound of it, and speaking allegorically, I said I felt that the brain of a person who needed Dilantin was like a bunch of dry twigs. It seemed that a thought of fear or anger would light the dry twigs, the fire would spread out of control, and the thoughts couldn't be turned off. Dilantin seemed to act like a gentle rain on the twigs, and the fire (and thoughts) could be kept under control.

I asked Peter if these impressions made sense. Peter said he had not done specific work with PHT, but my impressions were not inconsistent with the known fact that PHT prevented the spread of excessive electrical discharge. That was good news.

* * *

A few weeks after our last meeting, Peter performed an invaluable service. He sent me a copy of Goodman & Gilman's *Pharmacological Basis of Therapeutics,* considered to be the bible of pharmaceuticals by the medical profession, and said he thought I would find it useful.

I hadn't known there was such a book. In the section on PHT I found this:

> Coincident with the decrease in seizures there occurs improvement in intellectual performance. Salutary effects of the drug PHT on personality, memory, mood, cooperativeness, emotional stability, amenability to discipline, etc., are also observed, sometimes independently of seizure control.

I read and reread this paragraph. I could hardly believe it. Salutary effects in mood, emotional stability, etc. Here it was—in a medical book of high repute. Yet none of the doctors I'd met had ever heard of these uses. How could this be?

6.
A SOFT VOICE
IN A DEAF EAR

The time had come to tell the story to the medical profession. I had seen seven persons benefit from PHT, the electrical thoughts had been checked out and were not implausible, and there was the medical support of the Goodman & Gilman excerpt.

Now that the time had come, I didn't know how to proceed. I had always assumed that if I had enough evidence I would just "turn it over to the medical profession." That would be no problem, I thought. Now, faced with turning it over, I realized there was no "receiving department" in the medical profession—and I didn't know where to go. Dr. Silbermann and I discussed this problem at length and finally came up with what seemed a sensible plan.

Max, an associate professor at Columbia Presbyterian, was a personal friend of Dean H. Houston Merritt. This was the Merritt of Putnam and Merritt who had discovered that PHT was useful for epilepsy. What could be more logical than to bring the story to Dr. Merritt and Presbyterian Hospital?

At Max's suggestion we invited Dr. Merritt to have dinner at my home. Dr. Merritt accepted and brought with him Dr. Lawrence C. Kolb, Chief of Psychiatric Research at Presbyterian.

Since this was the first opportunity I'd had to present the PHT story in some detail, I was anxious to have other physicians present, and I invited my family physician, Dr. Alfred Steiner, and Dr. Ernest Klarch, a psychiatrist, whom Max had consulted in one of the seven cases. Also at dinner was my friend Sol. He had come from Miami so that the physicians could hear about PHT from a person other than myself.

Sol and I related our experiences with PHT. Then I told the physicians about the other five cases, and reported my observations of the medicine's effects on anger, fear, and the turned-on mind. They didn't express skepticism, but I think that the story, coming from a layman, was hard for them to believe. I was glad I could conclude with the quote from the respected medical source, Goodman & Gilman. To repeat:

> Salutary effects of PHT on personality, memory, mood, cooperativeness, emotional stability, amenability to discipline, etc., are also observed, sometimes independently of seizure control.

Dr. Merritt appeared surprised by this excerpt from Goodman & Gilman. He said he hadn't heard of it but hoped it was true. Then he suggested that maybe Presbyterian could do a study. Dr. Kolb agreed and said it could be arranged.

I couldn't let Dr. Merritt get away without asking him about possible side effects of PHT. He said that PHT had been in use for about twenty years, and a good record of safety had been established. There were side effects but they were rarely serious. He said PHT was non-habit-forming, and unlike many other substances it was not sedative in therapeutic doses. This was good news and I thanked Dr. Merritt. At the end of the meeting Dr. Kolb said he would be in touch with me.

Postscript to the dinner. When I'd invited Dr. Steiner and Dr. Klarch, appreciating their time was valuable, I said they could bill me for it. Dr. Steiner didn't send a bill. Dr. Klarch (fictitious name) sent a bill for $500. This seemed high. His only contribution to the meeting had been "Please pass the butter."

A few days after the meeting, Dr. Kolb phoned and told me he had arranged for Dr. Sidney Malitz to conduct the study. Dr. Malitz and I had dinner, and I repeated the PHT story. He said he was surprised to hear such a plausible story from a layman; he hadn't expected it. Apparently Dr. Kolb hadn't told him much about our discussion.

Dr. Malitz told me that he would set up two studies and I could fund them for $5,000 each. I said the matter was so urgent that I'd prefer to give $10,000 for each study, and this was agreed upon. I told Dr. Malitz I would appreciate it if he would keep me in close touch with how things were going. I didn't ask how the studies would be conducted; it didn't seem proper. But I had the feeling that much of my responsibility to PHT was now in the hands of professionals.

Alas. Week after week went by without my hearing from Dr. Malitz and a head of steam built up in me. When I finally called him after three months, I regret that I said, "Why the hell haven't I heard from you? You know how important this is." I don't think Sidney liked this opening remark and I can't say I blame him. He explained that the patients he had selected for the study were used to getting medicine three times a day, and since I'd only suggested 100 mg of Dilantin (one capsule) he was wondering if Parke-Davis could make it in smaller dosages, so it could be given three times a day. This excuse was so lame it needed crutches. Apparently Sidney had so little faith in PHT that he didn't think it could help unless the patients were psychologically influenced, and he hadn't even tried it. Further, if he'd looked into it, he would have found that Parke-Davis already made it in smaller dosages—a breakable 50 mg Infatab, a 30 mg capsule, and a liquid. After explaining to Dr. Malitz the different forms Dilantin came in, I expressed the hope that the study would now move forward.

Four more long months went by. I called Dr. Malitz again and this time, in the quietest way, asked him how things were going. He told me the study hadn't gotten started yet because he hadn't been able to get a placebo from Parke-Davis. I thanked him politely, and hung up with a heavy heart. Maybe Dr. Malitz couldn't get a placebo from Parke-Davis in seven months, but in those days most drugstores could supply a placebo in forty-eight hours.

In a last futile attempt I met with Dr. Kolb. He defended Dr. Malitz and said it was better to proceed slowly and carefully than the other way around. I didn't even argue with this platitude—it was such nonsense. Seven months had been wasted and I was discouraged. I'd taken what I thought was my best shot and hadn't got any results at all—not even negative.

Occasionally it may seem to the reader that I'm being critical of others. This is the opposite of my intention; I have too many motes in my own eye. But sometimes things have to be spelled out—otherwise this story would be too hard to believe. Looking back, it's easy to understand the position Dr. Malitz was in. He had been taught to think of PHT as an anticonvulsant. The idea that it had other uses came from an implausible source, a layman, and that didn't make it any easier for him. He undoubtedly had other research projects to which he gave priority—and PHT got on a back burner.

On other fronts things had not stood still. I had continued to send friends and acquaintances to doctors for trials with PHT. The effects were prompt and similar to those of the earlier cases. The numbers were mounting up. By now there were about twenty-five cases. In addition, I had a new source of information.

Dr. A. Lester Stepner, of Miami, had treated one of the first six people I'd seen take PHT. He had been so impressed with the results that he tried PHT with other patients. In a letter of April 1965, he summarized the cases of twelve patients he'd treated with PHT. In eleven of the twelve (he was unable to follow up the twelfth) he found PHT effective in treating anxiety, depression, anger, impulsiveness, temper outbursts, and incoherent thinking.

Coming at this time, Dr. Stepner's observations were a big psychological help to me, but they didn't seem to mean much to Dr. Silbermann and others I spoke to. I was beginning to understand the French phrase *idée fixe*.

The evidence was growing, but my confidence that I could convey it to others was shrinking. For months I had been buttonholing any doctor I ran into and informally talking about PHT. I must have spoken to a dozen of them during this period. None of them had heard of PHT being used for anything other than epilepsy. They were all (with one exception) polite, even kind, but they didn't give me any encouragement. That one doctor looked at me the way a Great Dane looks at a cricket and explained: "Medicine is a complicated matter, and I'd advise you to stick to Wall Street." Bless his heart.

I called a council of peace with my friends who knew of my interest in PHT. These friends were Dr. Max Silbermann, Dr. Peter Suckling, Yura Arkus-Duntov, and Howard Stein. We met in my office in early 1965 to decide the best way to get our information to the medical profession. For the first half of the meeting, we went over many cases in detail. By this time both Howard and Yura had each seen persons benefit from PHT, and we discussed how consistent our observations were with those reported in Goodman & Gilman.

We tape-recorded the meeting. Reading the transcript brings back those days in a lively way—I can still feel the warmth of my frustrations. There wasn't a suggestion I would make that Peter, Max, or Yura couldn't find an objection to. Toward the end I must have worn through my daily supply of PHT because I was hopping up and down with frustration.

The transcript of the meeting remembers better than I do. Here are a few excerpts:

> JACK: The problem before us is to awaken the doctors in the country to the potential of Dilantin. We're not in this for financial reasons, and we're not in it for glory. It's almost a crime not to try to get this information to the doctors. . . . We've got a lot of cases and we could do a thorough job of writing them up. If Dr. Silbermann would be willing . . .
>
> DR. MAX S: Jack, that would not be accepted by any medical journal. You could publish that at your own expense, there's no law against it.

JACK: Why wouldn't this be accepted by a medical journal?

DR. MAX S: Because. You know the old story. There is no blind control, and no medical journal would accept any drug study unless . . .

DR. PETER S: Unless you have had a computer in on it.

JACK: Max, are you serious? This can't be so.

YURA AND DR. MAX S: Oh, yes this is so.

JACK: Yura, we are talking about research, right? Please listen before you say no.

None of these people who took PHT knew each other. As far as they were concerned the study was blind. I asked them to write me letters that included details of their experiences. The same results from PHT are reported over and over again. This reinforces the evidence.

DR. PETER S: It is not accepted as proof and there's a devastating word that is applied to it, called anecdotal evidence. It doesn't go.

YURA: It's indirect proof.

JACK: Sorry fellows. Nobody in the room is thinking. These individuals wouldn't know which way to lie if they wanted to. They didn't know each other.

DR. PETER S: No, no. It's not that. This is the way . . .

JACK: Please. Let's not move the medical people all the way down to diapers. At least keep them in rompers, okay? I'm saying that if we added the Goodman & Gilman to Dr. Stepner's observations and the evidence of our twenty-five cases, write it up carefully, it's got to be received. We won't say we discovered America or anything like that. You, Dr. Silbermann, have got to make the effort.

DR. MAX S: Well, if we write it up and I publish it under my name and I send it in, no medical journal will accept it.

JACK: All right, Max, then no medical journal will accept it. At least we can send the information to the heads of the hospitals and say, "It would be a sin if we didn't tell you what we've found. Evaluate it on the basis of your own experience and do what you want." Once we've told the

heads of fifty hospitals, at least part of it should be off
our conscience. Let the non-use of it rest on other people's consciences . . .
   I don't care if machines are not involved. I can get
machines that will lie like anybody else. Will that help?
[I wouldn't have done that—in those days I was over
eighty percent honest.]
YURA: No, Jack. We are talking about the best means to
achieve this.

This discussion seems funny now, but it was very real
then. I was too near my own suffering and I was impatient
to get PHT to others. This impatience stayed with me, but
after bumping into enough brick walls and closed minds, I
realized it got in the way, and tabled it—with the help of
PHT. Without PHT I'd have had an implosion.
   For several weeks after the meeting, I thought about
what was said. I had argued with my friends at the top of
my lungs. But I knew they had my best interests at heart,
and I had to pay attention to them because they had experience where I had none.
   In the course of business I saw Howard Stein almost
every day. Every once in a while Howard would say, "If
you want to get anything done, you've got to do it your-
self." I didn't even respond to this remark at first. But
about the fourth time I heard it, I said, "Why are you per-
secuting me with that cliché?" He said, "I'm not using it
as a cliché; I mean it." "How can I do this myself?" I
asked. "I don't have any medical background, and besides
I have other dishes to wash, like the Dreyfus Fund and
Dreyfus & Co."
   But Howard said, "You'll see."

7.
ESTABLISHING A
MEDICAL FOUNDATION—

and the Story of My Life
(the Best Parts Left Out)

When I started to do well in business, I established a small foundation, the Dreyfus Charitable Foundation, for the purpose of giving money to what seemed good causes. It was my hope to be generally helpful, and the foundation gave money to numerous organizations and contributed equally to Protestant, Catholic, and Jewish charities. The responsibility of how to spend the money was left to these organizations.

But now I wanted to take over the responsibility of spending this money—I felt it should be spent on PHT research. PHT would need all the money I had been contributing and more, so I had to discontinue my usual contributions. And I could do this with a clear conscience—if the work on PHT was successful there would be many sources of charitable inquiry that would be helped by it. Consistent with this thinking, in 1965 the Dreyfus Charitable Foundation was changed into the Dreyfus Medical Foundation.

A medical foundation needs a medical director—but such a person can be difficult to obtain. Good physicians are fully occupied with their own matters and not easily sidetracked by what might seem a will-o'-the-wisp. After several months of search, Dr. Suckling introduced me to

Dr. William J. Turner, a neuropsychiatrist at Central Islip Hospital on Long Island.

At the first meeting with Dr. Turner I got a fine impression of him, and it's never changed. He said he had been anxious to meet with me because he had seen a number of persons, with disorders other than epilepsy, respond to Dilantin. We had several long discussions. After thinking about it for a few weeks Dr. Turner decided to join the Foundation as Medical Director.

At that time I thought that the Foundation would be able to achieve its goals within two or three years. It seemed unwise for Dr. Turner to break his connections with Central Islip Hospital and move to New York City, so he joined us as Director on a part-time basis. Bill took a small office near his home in Huntington, Long Island, hired a secretary and medical assistant, and we were in business. (Jumping ahead a few years—when it became apparent that my timetable was optimistic, I was fortunate in being able to persuade Dr. Samuel Bogoch, a professor at the Boston University School of Medicine and Chairman of the International Institute for the Brain Sciences, to join the Foundation on a full-time basis as General Director; Dr. Turner continued as Director.)

At the outset, Dr. Turner and I had the objective of proving—or disproving—that PHT was more than an anticonvulsant. We were as open to negative possibilities as to positive ones. I had my ideas as to what we would find: but if they were wrong, I didn't want to spend my time trying to prove something that wasn't so—there are pleasanter ways of making a fool of oneself.

Our plan was simple. The Foundation would sponsor a few studies at medical institutions. My guess was that this might take $150,000 to $200,000 a year for the next two or three years. If these studies were successful, the facts about PHT would then be in the hands of professionals. Once this happened I thought the word would spread like wildfire throughout the medical profession, and the job would be done. If I had been told, then, that in the next fifteen years the Foundation was going to spend over $15 million* (and the job not completed), I wouldn't have believed it. One reason is that $15 million was three times as much money as I had at that time.

Talking about money in connection with this work is awkward for me. I don't want to sound like I think I'm a boy scout. But there is a point to be made here. If I hadn't been lucky enough to have the money, I wouldn't have gotten to first base.

When I think back to my first job, at $15 a week, I realize what an implausible person I was to have a lot of money. Implausible is too weak a word. I'll tell how it happened. If you believe in fate, or whatever, you're entitled to believe the money was given to me to spend on PHT.

When I was a boy my parents were not poor, nor were they rich. Once, my father, who sold candy wholesale, was out of a job and down to his last two weeks of spending money for the family. But that was his low point, and I wasn't even aware of it at the time.

When I was ten years old, I learned what money was for. The laws of Montgomery, Alabama, permitted me to go to the movies by myself at that age. My parents would give me a dime on Saturday mornings, and the Strand Theater was assured of an early customer. I would see the Pathé News, the "To Be Continued Next Saturday" serial, and a movie—sometimes twice. After the movie, when I

* By now, 1988, over $60 million

had a nickel slipped to me by one of my uncles, I would go to Franco's and buy a long hotdog with sauerkraut and red sauce. They were especially delicious since my dear mother considered them poisonous.

The first time the thought of making a living came up was when I was fifteen. At that time I played golf in Montgomery with a boy of my age, Alan Rice. We were both good golfers; I played a little better than he did but he didn't think so—this miscalculation kept me in quarters. One day, while at the seventh-hole water fountain, Alan, a serious boy, said that someday he was going to make $100,000. When that happened, that was going to be it! He was going to retire and live on the income of $5,000 a year. Alan's father was a storekeeper, and I figured Alan must have heard this from him. I was impressed, or I wouldn't have remembered it to this day. I knew I'd never make that much money. But if a miracle happened and I made $100,000, there'd be two retirees.

When I was sixteen, my father had enough money to send me to college, Lehigh University. I studied the minimum and got a C average—my only A was in music appreciation, and my only distinction was that I was captain of the golf team. At college my brain didn't come to grips with the problem of how I would earn a living; it didn't occur to me to study something practical. It's just as well. Lehigh is a fine engineering school; if I'd fooled with that, I would have flunked out. Even as it was, for a year after graduation I had nightmares that they took my diploma back.

When I got out of college I didn't know what I wanted to do. Well really, I guess I did, but I didn't discuss it with my father. What I wanted to do was to not work. Sometimes I had this nice fantasy. I thought if I had the courage (I wasn't even close) I'd ask John D. Rockefeller for $1 million. My reason was that he was too old to thoroughly enjoy his money, and I wasn't too old to thoroughly enjoy his money. I could play golf, travel, and be happy in every way, and he could enjoy this—secondhand.

If the reader has gotten the impression that I lacked enthusiasm for work he is on the right track. However, I had to get a job. I tried selling insurance and couldn't stand it. Everybody I said hello to was a prospect. I worked on my first potential customer for two months and must have played golf with him a dozen times (he couldn't hit the ball out of his own shadow) and finally got up enough courage to try to sell him an annuity. He turned me down. I went out to the street and cried—and retired from the insurance business. Money earned in insurance: zero.

My next effort was in the candy business. My father thought that maybe I could help him in sales. By then we had moved to New York. He was concentrating on selling candy to just a few large customers, the chain stores— Woolworth's, Kress, McCrory, and others. To help me learn the business, he got me a job in a candy factory, Edgar P. Lewis, of Malden, Massachusetts. I liked making candy, and for six months worked on the marmalade slab, making imitation orange slices, and barely lifting 100-pound bags of sugar into a boiling cauldron. In the late afternoon I'd go back to my boarding house and take a nap before dinner. Those were solid naps. When I woke up I didn't know where I was or what I was.

My salary at Edgar P. Lewis was $15 a week—and I lived on it. No hardship, but not luxurious either. Room and board was $10.50 (lunch excluded). Both breakfast and dinner had the advantage of baked beans. I had one luxury (a necessity in getting to work), an old Buick my father had given me. Garage used up a buck a week. That didn't leave much out of the $15. When I was on double dates with Mat Suvalsky, an old college friend, Mat was encouraged to split the gas with me. A happy period in my life. But I wasn't any closer to my fortune—the Alan Rice $100,000.

After six months my father felt that I had eaten enough candy and I was ready for sales training with him. My specific chores were to drive the car and carry the samples; and I would listen while my father talked to the candy buyers. I remember the first meeting I attended. While candy was being discussed I toyed with a fountain pen on the buyer's desk. When we got to the street my hand went into my pocket and, to my surprise, came out with the fountain pen. My father was not elated.

Well, we struggled along for a few months, but you know how it is with father and son, they don't always work well together. Besides, I guess selling wasn't my racket. My father had always impressed on me how important the other man's time was, and I think he overdid it. So I retired from the candy business and still needed a job.

We hear about those people who, while still playing with their rattles, know exactly what they want to do in life. Well, I was twenty-two and I'd never had any idea what I wanted to do. Naturally I got in the doldrums. My parents were patient—my mother was the sweetest person I've ever known—and they didn't push me. I lay around the apartment on West 88th Street, played bridge in the afternoon and evening, and fell asleep around 3 A.M. listening to Clyde McCoy playing "Sugar Blues." My father, who was tough on me but loved me, thought I should see a psychiatrist. And I did, twice a week.

During this period an uncle got me a job with an industrial designer. Salary, $18 a week. The designer insisted I wear a hat, a Homburg no less; this purchase ate up my excess profits. I accompanied my employer to different stores he represented, with the thought that sooner or later I would catch on to the business. But I wasn't a quick learner. However, before I could get fired the designer offered to raise my salary from $18 a week to $50 a week, if I stopped seeing the psychiatrist, and he proposed we take a trip to Florida together. I was just bright enough to sense an ulterior motive, and resigned.

Insurance, candy, and industrial design—two strikes and a foul tip. Back to bridge, Clyde McCoy, and the psychiatrist. My parents were discouraged but they weren't surprised. My father always expected I'd have trouble making a living. I had no discernible useful aptitude, and my father had a suspicion that I was lazy (which suspicion he didn't keep from me). Privately, I agreed with him.

Anyway, lazy or not, I didn't have a job. One night at the bridge club one of the players, who knew I was indigent, said I might like the brokerage business. Wall Street was the last place I'd have thought of trying, and with reluctance kept an appointment he made. My father went with me to the garment district branch of Cohen, Simondson & Co., members of the New York Stock Exchange. I was interviewed by a customer's broker who needed an assistant to answer his phones and keep his charts. I got the job, $25 a week. I thought I got it on my good looks, but years later I learned that my father had paid the customer's broker twenty weeks' salary in advance.

This time I took an interest in a job. The fluctuating prices and the gamble of the stock market struck one of my aptitudes. And it wasn't hard looking at the pretty models in the garment district. In a week I felt so much better that I tendered my resignation to the psychiatrist. Six months later I passed a stock exchange test, and became a junior customer's broker.

Although I liked the stock market, I was no threat to make a fortune; part of the job was approaching people for business and I didn't like that—it was selling again. After several years with Cohen, Simondson, I applied for a job as a full customer's broker at Bache & Co., and got turned down. Then E. A. Pierce & Co., later Merrill Lynch, Pierce, Fenner & Bean, took a chance and gave me a job at $75 a week—which I didn't quite earn.

While at Merrill Lynch I met a spry, eighty-year-old partner of the firm, Almar Shatford. In those days I got the flu and colds a lot and, being from Alabama, bundled up in cold weather. Mr. Shatford advised me to cut out that nonsense and wear less clothing. The first year I just wore a topcoat and there was improvement. The next year I discarded the topcoat and didn't get a single cold. And there was a serendipitous effect. Till then, when I was late to work, Victor Cook, our managing partner, would give me a friendly unfriendly look. But now I had the edge on Victor. When I arrived late, without a topcoat, Vic couldn't be sure I wasn't returning from the men's room.

I wasn't what you'd call a hard worker. There was usually an hour for lunch at Wilfred's across the street, and when the market closed at three o'clock I was on my way to my real enjoyment, bridge at the Cavendish Club. At my peak I was no more than a mediocre customer's broker. In market judgment I was probably above average—my charts were a big help here—but in commissions for the firm I was a dud. My career high was a salary of $1,000 a month—and this was more than my friend Victor Cook ever expected of me.

Making a thousand a month must have unsettled my brain because, although classified 4-F, I volunteered for the Coast Guard. At Sheepshead Bay I worked my way steadily up through the ranks, to Seaman 2nd Class. The Coast Guard sifted through my talents, and put me in a high position—on top of a garbage wagon where I was third in charge. But enough of my wartime exploits.

From the Coast Guard I returned to Merrill Lynch and my job as a customer's broker. One afternoon, after playing gin at the City Athletic Club, Chester Gaines, a specialist on the floor of the New York Stock Exchange, said that judging by the way I played gin I'd do well trading on the floor, and should buy a seat. It was a good idea but the funds I had were a little short of the purchase price—about ninety-seven percent short.

In those days I used to play golf with a friend, Jerry Ohrbach, at Metropolis Country Club (let me brag and say I won the club championship seven years in a row). One day, when we were in the same foursome, I got a seven on the first hole, an easy par five. I was steaming, and asked Jerry what odds he would give against my getting a thirty-three on that nine. Par was thirty-five, so that meant I would have to be four under for the next eight holes. Jerry said 1,000-to-1. I said I'll take a hundred dollars worth of that if you like, and he said okay. He could afford the hundred thousand and I could afford the hundred dollars. Jerry had the best of the odds and I had a shot at my Alan Rice fortune. I made him sweat to the last hole. I needed a birdie there for the thirty-three, but didn't come close.

When Chester Gaines made the suggestion of the stock

exchange seat, I spoke to Jerry about it. He told me that the golf bet had scared him so much he would like to be partners with me. By borrowing from my father, one of my uncles, my wife, and adding my own few dollars, I got up twenty-five percent of the necessary capital. Jerry and his father, Nathan, put up the rest and became limited partners in the small firm, Dreyfus & Co., members of the New York Stock Exchange. And we lived happily ever after. Well, not quite.

Our back-office work was done by Bache & Co., the firm that had turned me down as a customer's broker. A friend of mine, John Behrens, handled my accounts in the office, and I went to the floor of the Exchange where I did two-dollar brokerage and traded for the firm's account. I liked the floor. It was a lot of walking—with a little thinking thrown in—and the hours of ten to three fitted well with my lazy bones.

In the first year, 1946, with capital of $100,000, we made $14,000 trading. Not as bad as you'd think—'46 was a bear market. A floor joke describes it, "The market was so bad that not even the liars made money." I don't think Nathan Ohrbach realized how well we did not to have lost our shirts. Nathan, who had the misfortune to walk into a brokerage office for the first time in 1929, had the indestructible opinion that you couldn't beat the market and was restless for Dreyfus & Co. to become a commission firm.

One day Jerry introduced me to one of the partners of the firm of Lewisohn & Sons. The capital partners wanted to retire, and Jerry and Nathan thought we should take over this old firm, stop clearing through Bache, and do our own back-office work. I mildly resisted—it didn't look like that good a deal, and besides it sounded like work. But I was told that three of the Lewisohn partners would remain and run the business, and I could stay on the floor. So I agreed.

We bought this turkey, with trimmings. The Ohrbachs and I got the trimmings. The excuse the capital partners had given for wanting to retire was that they were getting older. Even if they had been getting younger it would have been a good idea.

Without going into the reasons, it wasn't long before I had to leave the floor, where I was reasonably competent, and take on managing a brokerage firm, where I wasn't competent at all. Nathan Ohrbach soon found there were more ways of losing money on Wall Street than trading in the market. Our capital went down rapidly—mine vanished—and it looked like I was going to make my Alan Rice fortune in reverse. We couldn't even go out of business easily, and decided to try to stick it out. The Ohrbachs were good about it and drew no interest on their money. I cut my salary to zero, and we struggled along.

After a while business got so good we broke even. The Ohrbachs and I thought we should advertise, and we set aside $20,000 of hard (unearned) money for the purpose. In those days one agency handled all the Wall Street advertising, and it was dreary. I thought we should try another agency.

At that time the firm of Doyle, Dane, and Bernbach was in swaddling clothes. The partners were friends of the Ohrbachs and agreed to handle our account. But for our budget they couldn't afford to write the copy. So I had to. To my great surprise I loved it; it was an aptitude that had been hidden from me. Our account executive, Freddie

Dossenbach, and I used to have lunch at a corner table next to a window at Schwartz's on Broad Street. Inspired by Swiss cheese and liverwurst, with iced tea, I'd write copy to fit Freddie's cartoons. The ads were so different from what was being done on Wall Street that we got a lot of attention for the money being spent. Business got better and the firm started to grow. Soon we had enough partners to always have a quorum for an argument.

One day the Dreyfus Fund walked through the front door and we didn't know it. A fine gentleman, John Nesbett, applied for a position. John was the sole proprietor of a $600,000 mutual fund, the Nesbett Fund. He had struggled with it for several years, but with a management fee of $3,000 a year it had become impractical for him to continue. When John joined Dreyfus & Co. the name of his fund was changed to the Dreyfus Fund, and we took over the struggle. In the next five years Dreyfus & Co. lost about a million and a half dollars of its earnings on the Fund. During that period I got looks from some of my partners that at best could be called askance. But one day the fund started to break even. From then on it became a winner.

I made money in the stock market, a great deal of it in Polaroid stock. Did I carefully screen the list to select this stock? No. I wouldn't even have known there was such a company if I hadn't had a brother-in-law who worked there. I bought the stock initially for the wrong reason— Polaroid's 3-D glasses—and made money because of the camera.

It would appear I had some luck. The Ohrbachs pushed me into the commission business, the Dreyfus Fund walked into the office, and I bought the right stock for the wrong reason. As I said earlier I was an implausible person to have made a lot of money.

In the late 1960s I retired from my businesses. Since then I have worked full time with the Dreyfus Medical Foundation.

* * *

The newly established Dreyfus Medical Foundation funded its first study in 1966—with hope, and $57,000. It was a dud. It could be called a waste of time and money. But that wouldn't be quite right—it was part of education. I was learning how difficult it was to develop anyone's interest in PHT. As to the study, I'll make it brief. And I'll skip names. As explained earlier, complaining is not one of the purposes of this book.

Dr. Turner introduced me to members of the staff of a large hospital in the metropolitan area. They said they were interested in PHT and had a good patient population for conducting a study. I explained what had happened in the previous study—I didn't want to make that sort of mistake again—and said I'd like to be present in the early stages of the work. My experience, unsophisticated as it was, might be useful. They agreed to this and asked for $57,000 for the study.

I'd been given the impression that the study would start without delay, but it wasn't for several months that I was invited to attend the first interview with patients, conducted by Dr. Blank.

Four patients were interviewed in my presence. To my dismay, I was not allowed to say a word to these patients, although I sat just a few feet from them. If I wanted to ask a question, I had to write it on a slip of paper and hand it to Dr. Blank. Using "local mail" didn't improve my ability to communicate with these patients. One case is worth mentioning, a man who said he jackknifed in bed at night. Dr. Blank didn't ask for particulars, but I did—by note— and learned that several times each night, before he fell asleep, the patient's legs would jerk up almost to his head. I was surprised that PHT had not already been tried with him—these involuntary movements seemed a form of convulsion. After the session I expressed the opinion to Dr. Blank that three of the four patients were good candidates for PHT. I was never told whether they were given it— there was an air of mystery about everything—but I don't think they were.

The upshot of this study was that, two years later, the physician in charge of the study made the vapid statement at a medical meeting that "more work was needed in this field." Well, you couldn't argue with that.

It's hard to realize how frustrating this was. Here I was, eager to give money for studies on an established medicine, and couldn't find the right people to give it to.

* * *

One fine day, in 1966, Dr. Turner asked me if I'd like to participate in the conduct of a study. I told him I'd like to, but I didn't know it was possible. Bill said he thought it could be arranged. A few weeks later Bill made arrangements through a friend of his, Dr. Oscar Resnick of the Worcester Foundation, for that foundation and ours to conduct a joint study at the Worcester County Jail.

Bill and I visited Dr. Resnick at his home in Worcester, Massachusetts, the following Sunday. On both sides of a nice lunch we discussed the proposed study. Until Bill had brought up the subject, I'd never thought about a study in a prison. After all a prison is not a hospital and doesn't necessarily have sick people. But now that I thought about it, it seemed that nervous conditions could be a contributing cause in many criminal acts, particularly those of anger and violence. I discussed this with Dr. Resnick, who had done many studies at this jail. He agreed and said he thought we'd find an ample number of people who had problems with their nerves.

When we discussed how the interview with the prisoners should be conducted, Oscar won a lifelong friendship with me when he said, "Look, Jack, you know what you're looking for. It'll be a lot easier if you ask the questions. I'll chime in when I think it's necessary."

This jail study was to be an unusual experience for me —in some ways the most fruitful of my life.

8.
ELEVEN ANGRY MEN

In 1966 Dr. Resnick and I conducted a study on the effects of PHT with prisoners at the Worcester County Jail in Massachusetts. It was done on a double-blind crossover basis. Helping us with the study was Ms. Barbara Homan, medical assistant to Dr. Turner.

The Worcester County Jail was a "short-term" jail. Although some of the inmates had committed serious crimes, no one sentenced to more than eighteen months was sent there.

From the outside the jail looked like an ordinary building. On the inside, except in the cell area, it resembled an old high school. For our work we were assigned a small room with a nice window on the second floor. This room was plainly furnished but comfortable, with a long table and some chairs. Liaison with the prisoners was handled by Lt. William D'Orsay, a kind and well-liked man.

Drug studies were not uncommon at the jail.* It was the custom for these studies to be done with volunteers, paid a dollar a day. We followed custom. Ms. Homan did preliminary screening of forty-two volunteers, and eliminated twenty of the least likely candidates. This left

---

* Clearance for the study was given by the warden, Sheriff Joseph Smith, and Dr. Cyrus Paskevitch, the prison physician.

twenty-two volunteers for Dr. Resnick and me to interview.

These twenty-two volunteers were interviewed carefully. This was a study of individuals, not prisoners; we had no intention of giving PHT to anyone just because he was in prison. We were looking for individuals who had symptoms we thought would respond to PHT. Among the most important of these symptoms were: excessive anger, excessive fear, and an overbusy mind that was difficult to turn off.

After two days of interviews, eleven prisoners were selected. Most of them had participated in other drug studies and didn't expect to get a medicine that would actually help them. They thought we were doing the study for our own purposes and they had volunteered mainly to ease their boredom. When we told them that we wanted only the truth about what the medicine did, they expressed skepticism that it would do anything. This attitude was good—it minimized the possibility of their being psychologically influenced.

In the initial interviews I was glad I was not alone in the room with a few of the prisoners. There was an animalistic bristle about them you could feel. One man had eyes with a yellowish glow that reminded me of an ocelot I'd seen. After a few interviews, whether because of PHT or getting to know them better, I felt comfortable with all the prisoners.

Dr. Resnick left most of the questioning of the prisoners to me. I tried to keep the interviews comfortable and friendly. This seemed to help the subjects relax and they spoke freely. Some of them were more expressive than others, but communication was good with all of them.

Procedure. The eleven prisoners chosen for the study were interviewed for a second time, this time intensively. As specifically as we could, we got an inventory of their symptoms and complaints. Then they were placed on PHT (100 mg in the morning and 50 mg in the afternoon) and were not told what to expect of the medicine. They were interviewed several hours after the initial dose, the next day, and again at the end of a week.

Remarkable improvement in symptoms was observed. To see if similar results would be obtained under the most objective circumstances, we decided to do a double-blind, crossover to single-blind, study.

To do such a study it was desirable to approximate the original conditions. We thought this could be achieved by taking the prisoners off PHT for a week. However, when they were interviewed at the end of the week, their general condition was better than when we had first met them. It was as though the week on PHT had been a vacation from their nerves and the benefits had carried forward. We had to wait a second week before the original conditions were approximated.

Before starting the double-blind study we explained the procedure to the prisoners. Some of them would receive PHT, others an inert substance called a placebo. The capsules would be identical in appearance—the prisoners wouldn't know what they contained and we wouldn't know, thus "double-blind." Then they would be interviewed as before: a few hours after the first pill, after a night's sleep, and a week later. At that time we would make our decision as to which of them had received PHT, and which placebo.

What we did not tell the prisoners was that when this

decision had been made, those subjects we thought had been on placebo would be placed on "single-blind." They would be given PHT without being told it was PHT. In that way, further non-subjective evidence would be obtained.

Summary

We were correct in our assessment of ten of the prisoners on the double-blind. We were incorrect in one. The unusual circumstances in this case explain why.*

In the study it was observed that the eleven prisoners had many symptoms in common that responded to PHT. Among these symptoms in common were restlessness, irritability, fear, anger, inability to concentrate, poor mood, lack of energy, sleeping problems, and an overactive brain.

Symptoms not common to all prisoners, such as headache, stomach distress, chest pain, muscular pain, skin rash, and dizziness, disappeared while the subjects were on PHT and reappeared when it was withdrawn.

This study was recorded on tape with the prisoners' permission. Transcribed, there are 605 pages covering 130 interviews.†

The results were exceptional. Brief summaries of the

---

* In the early part of the study, Danny R.'s response to PHT was similar to that of the other prisoners. During the control part of the study, Danny R. got news that made him think his daughter was going blind. He didn't tell us, and we misassessed his realistic nervousness and decided he was on placebo. (For details, see Appendix, p. 159.)

† An 80-page condensation is available in limited number for those interested. The 605-page transcript is on file at the Dreyfus Medical Foundation.

eleven cases are included in this book. Only four are included here. Please see the other seven in Appendix.

JAMES L.

Before PHT:

I feel miserable, a bunch of nerves.

I have a grudge on me I can't get rid of . . . I take it out on everyone. It's so bad that sometimes I have myself locked in so I won't cause any trouble.

I can't work or nothing. When you're down-and-out there isn't much you can do.

I can't digest my food right . . . I don't feel like eating nothing.

My thinking is bad, there are quite a few thoughts in my mind, I can't concentrate at all. It takes me a day and a half to write one letter.

I get them phantom limb pains [he had a wooden leg] quite a bit, at least three times a week. The pain, I can just take so much of it. I can't sleep and I can't sit still or nothing.

Sometimes I have them headaches in the afternoon and at night I get them right back again.

With PHT (Non-Blind):

I feel a lot better. All the guys down there say I ain't the same guy . . . because I let them all out of their cells. [James L. was a trusty.] I didn't lock nobody up.

Now I'm eating like a fool, before I couldn't eat.

I get them headaches once in a while but not too often. That's why I stopped taking those aspirins.

After Being Off PHT (Two Weeks):

I never get to sleep . . . I sleep about an hour, that's all.

I get weak but I can't seem to hold my weight. The guys put me on the bed and I come out of it after a while.

I get them headaches quite often now. I'm getting phantom limb pains again . . . I had it again yesterday. I couldn't even lay down on the bed. I kept twisting and turning.

I'll read a story and, as a matter of fact, I won't even know what I read.

With Placebo (Double-Blind):

I'm down and out right now. My mind's all bunched up now. I passed out Wednesday. I get headaches.

Anger, about the same as it was before the pills.

I had those phantom limb pains Wednesday.

With PHT (Single-Blind):

I feel good right now . . . I feel altogether different . . . I feel much better since I got them pills.

I've been kidding around with everybody . . . For the last two days the fellows have been saying I'm not the same guy. No headaches. No phantom limb pains.

DAVID H.

Before PHT:

I have a temper that shouldn't be . . . I shake when I'm angry and can't stop. I have stomach trouble . . . I think it's from nerves.

If something happens, I twist and turn it in my mind until I've made a problem out of nothing . . . I can't turn my mind off. I can't go to sleep.

Quite often I'll get depressed and start worrying about home and what's going on outside these lovely walls. I lose all hope and energy.

With PHT:

Well, I feel I'm a lot calmer . . . I can sit still, without jumping up.

For the past five or six days I've been sure of myself in the things I say and what I do. I get angry just as fast but I can control it . . . it doesn't keep poppin' back into my mind.

I used to read three or four chapters without knowing what I read. Now I can lie there and remember what I've read.

I've been eating my meals and enjoying them.

After Being Off PHT (Two Weeks):

I feel very tired, irritable and grouchy. I'm not getting along well . . . People are getting on my nerves to the extent where I'm ready to assassinate them.

I don't eat hardly anything . . . I'm not sleeping very well . . . I feel just terrible.

I got a few problems and I just can't get them out of my mind. I'm worrying about them all the time . . . I've tried my case a thousand times.

With PHT (Double-Blind):

I think I'm on the Dilantin right now. I'm not nervous . . . I'm not tense or ready to jump at anyone.

I'm not grouchy . . . I seem to still have a temper, but I go into a situation with a little more confidence. I don't just jump off the handle.

I seem able to push my thoughts aside . . . read a couple of stories and know what I read.

I feel fine as far as my stomach goes . . . My appetite has picked up . . . I been sleeping better . . . able to go right to sleep.

CLIFFORD S.

Before PHT:

I'm very highstrung . . . I let everything build up inside . . . Then I just explode. I do a lot of thinking.

I get these wicked headaches . . . I'll take six or seven

aspirin . . . and the headache won't go away. I'll have it all day.

I don't sleep well. Between twelve and two in the morning I usually get these nightmares . . . scare a guy right out of his head.

With PHT:

I just feel wonderful . . . You know how I can feel my nerves are relaxed? I've done four paintings; I don't paint when I'm nervous because I can't concentrate . . . If I can sit down and do a painting a day it makes me happy.

I'm in a good mood. I don't feel angry at anybody . . . I've only really got mad once since the last time I seen you. It went right away.

I've been sleeping a lot. I ain't jumpy all the time. I ain't looking behind me anymore.

After Being Off PHT (Two Weeks):

I'm tense inside, I can't stay in one place too long, I get up and move around . . . I just pick a book up, look at it and throw it back down.

I feel that anger . . . Whenever I get in a fight I can't control myself.

I wake up about five or six times during the night.

With Placebo (Double-Blind):

My nerves are jittery inside . . . I can't sit in one place too long.

This week when I was lifting, I got dizzy three or four times and I was only working out with light weights.

I know my mind's always been going on. Actually, I don't feel these pills have done anything for me.

With PHT (Single-Blind):

I just feel good. I am completely relaxed . . . I ain't nervous, tense or nothing.

There's no anger at all.

Sleep better . . . ain't tired . . . all kinds of energy; washing windows, floors. I can concentrate better.

PHILIP B.

Before PHT:

I am quite nervous now. I've been more or less nervous all my life. And shake a lot, you just feel it, that you're shaking.

If I get nervous my hands break out in a little rash. I get tightness in my chest quite often. It's a pain, it takes your breath away sometimes.

I think a lot, there is too much on my mind. I try to put it out of my mind and it just stays there. The mind wanders and it doesn't focus on what I'm doing. Sometimes it's three o'clock in the morning before I get to sleep.

With PHT:

I feel good all over now. I seem to relax a lot more. Since I've been taking the pills I haven't been walking around, pacing back and forth so much. These past few nights I've been going right to sleep.

I haven't been so depressed. I've been eating better. And I haven't had those pains in my chest. And I can concentrate better on my work and I'm not making as many mistakes.

After Being Off PHT (Two Weeks):

Well, I feel I'm right back where I was before I started taking the pills. I don't sleep well. I walk around all the time. Nervous all the time—agitated, quick-tempered, get shook up.

I'm always thinking—wandering away—always thinking of different things. I've been very depressed.

With PHT (Double-Blind):

I feel good, very good, feel a lot better, honestly. And I haven't had those chest pains this week at all. The rash

—it cleared right up. I'm more relaxed.

I can just forget about things now. I've been able to do my work better. The last few days I've been goin' to sleep right off. I feel much better than I have for the last three years.

Suggestions from the Prisoners for the Use of PHT in Prisons

When the study was over we met with the inmates as a group for the first time. Each of the prisoners had told us he wanted to continue taking PHT. But I learned this was not going to be permitted, and there was nothing I could do about that. But I could tell the prisoners what I knew about the medicine—it might be useful to them later on.

We had a long, friendly discussion. As we were saying goodbye John G. volunteered:

JOHN G: If this pill was ever put on the market it would be a godsend to both Walpole and Concord prisons. Judging by this group here, it'd work miracles up there. You have men doing ten, fifteen, twenty, and life. And that's where I'd like to see them back up a whole truckload of the stuff and—

JACK D: You mean Dilantin?

JOHN G: Dilantin is right. Those guys are walkin' on edge all the time. There's where the trouble starts, more so than here. These fellows are all going fairly short. Up there you got a bunch of fellows that got nothing to lose and, well, they're all packed in together.

JACK D: You think that in those prisons—

JOHN G: I think they need it even worse than the fellows do here. You can ask Jim and Spike.

JACK D: Do you agree with that, Spike?

VICTOR M: Oh, yes, I agree with that very much.

JACK D: What would you say, Jim?

JAMES L: The same thing. I was there for a while myself and I know. It would help a lot of them guys. You walk around there and if you say the wrong thing, you're liable to go bouncing off the wall.

JOHN G: Those guys are so on edge they gotta take yellow jackets and bennies once in a while to relieve that. What if they didn't have this tension built up? They wouldn't have the trouble they do now.

JACK D: Well, John, thank you for the thought.

The prisoners' suggestion that the use of PHT, on a voluntary basis, be permitted inside a prison should be considered. Some prisoners are in jail because of problems in their nervous systems, and these problems are exacerbated by their confinement. With too much time to think and brood, it's no wonder that some prisoners live in a sort of hell—and can't help imposing it on those around them. Allowing PHT to be taken on a voluntary basis could make an important difference to those individuals who need it— and to others who are endangered by their potential for violence. When one realizes that PHT is not habit-forming, withholding it from prisoners is the opposite of protection of their rights.

* * *

As stated earlier, this study was not of prisoners as such but a study of individuals with problems of their nervous sytems. The objective was to see if, in a double-blind study, the effects of PHT that had been observed on an uncontrolled basis would be confirmed. They were, and additional effects of PHT were observed.*

I felt the time had come to go to the Federal government.

* I participated in two further studies in institutions, one with Dr. Resnick at the Lyman Reformatory for Boys in Lyman, Massachusetts, the other at the Patuxent Institution in Maryland, with Dr. Joel Elkes, head of psychiatry at Johns Hopkins, and Dr. Joseph Stephens and Dr. Lino S. Covi, also of Hopkins. Although not controlled studies, the results were similar to those of the Worcester study. (See Appendix, p. 162.)

9.
TRAVELS
WITH THE GOVERNMENT

Few of us have a clear picture of the Federal government and how it operates. With millions of people in it, government has to be run by regulations. This leads to routine. Where there's routine, innovation doesn't thrive. I'm not being critical, government means well. But I'll tell you this, if you want the government to do something outside of routine—and expect to see it happen in your lifetime—you'd better arrange for reincarnation.

I didn't know this in 1966, and with the optimism of a boy scout I approached the Federal government. I would have gone to the government sooner but had felt the evidence was too informal. Now, with the jail study done, the time was right. I had two thoughts in mind. The first was that the government might take the matter off my hands. I hoped for this, but wasn't counting on it. My second thought was that I didn't want to do anything contrary to government policy. Their objectives and mine were the same. If I was to proceed on my own, I needed official advice.

There were two logical places to go: the Department of Health, Education and Welfare, and the Food and Drug Administration. Since I was a layman, the Department of Health seemed the appropriate place. At that time John W. Gardner was Secretary of H.E.W. It took me about a month to get an appointment with the Secretary. That seemed like a long time. When I got to know the government better I realized that a month was instantaneous.

I met with Secretary Gardner in Washington in May 1966. We talked for fifty minutes. That is, I talked for the first forty minutes and he talked for the last ten. In those forty minutes I summarized my experience with Dilantin and my observations of its benefits in others. I told him of my disappointment in the two hospital studies I'd sponsored, of setting up the Dreyfus Medical Foundation, and of the double-blind study at the Worcester County Jail.

Secretary Gardner listened. From the experience I'd had it wouldn't have surprised me if he had been skeptical. But he wasn't. The Secretary seemed to sense that I was on the right track. Although he didn't suggest that the government take a hand, he gave me three helpful suggestions.

The first suggestion had to do with my unmedical terminology. The Secretary laughed when I made my "dry twigs" analogy. He said he liked it but thought more sophisticated language would stand me in good stead in talking with physicians. Of course he was right, and now I talk of "post-tetanic potentiation" and "post-tetanic afterdischarge" as if they were old friends. His second suggestion was that I should tell Parke-Davis about my findings. I followed this suggestion, too, as will be explained later.

The third suggestion came as a surprise, but I welcomed it. The Secretary said I should seek national publicity for the story. He understood my disappointment with the lack of results from the two hospitals. However, he was sure that somewhere in the United States there were hospitals and physicians who would be interested in the story.

I told Secretary Gardner I could try *Life* magazine. A

few months earlier *Life* had done a kind article about me by Marshall Smith with the understated title, "Maverick Wizard Behind the Wall Street Lion." Marshall and I had become good friends, and I thought he might introduce me to *Life's* science department. The Secretary said that *Life* would be an excellent place for this story, if they would do it.

The meeting with Secretary Gardner was most helpful. His suggestions were good and I followed them all.

* * *

It wasn't easy to get *Life* magazine to do a medical article recommended by a layman. Albert Rosenfeld, *Life's* science editor, was understandably cautious. He had several sessions with me in which he listened carefully to the evidence. Then Al said he would like to do the story, but *Life* would require a medical event as a peg. He said a medical meeting would serve the purpose. Before making a firm commitment, however, Al wanted to get the reactions of a good friend, Dr. Joel Elkes, Director of Psychiatry at Johns Hopkins.

Before I met Dr. Elkes I thought of him as a hurdle. But after a discussion with him, I found I had a friend. Dr. Elkes said the subject was of particular interest since ten years earlier he had planned to do research on PHT with other physicians. But just at that time an exciting new medicine, thorazine, had appeared, and their interest had been sidetracked. Dr. Elkes was helpful in setting up the meeting that *Life* required, and in 1966 a symposium on PHT was held at the annual meeting of the American College of Neuropsychopharmacology.

In September 1967 *Life* published an article by Albert

Rosenfeld—"10,000-to-1 Payoff." The article was a turn-ing point. The response to it, and to the *Reader's Digest* condensation of it printed in thirteen languages, forced us to increase our small staff to keep up with phone calls and to answer letters. Many physicians wrote that they were using PHT for a variety of purposes.

We received thousands of letters from the public. The best side of human nature showed up. The writers ex-pressed deep appreciation for benefits they got from PHT as a result of the articles. Many described their experi-ences in detail in the hope that by so doing they might help others. We selected a hundred of these letters and made a booklet for physicians. But readership was poor; doctors consider letters "anecdotal."

The *Life* and *Reader's Digest* articles opened things up. Now there were institutions and individual physicians with genuine interest in doing work on PHT. Soon the Foundation was sponsoring over a dozen studies. We got as far from home base as Chichester, England. There, Dr. Lionel Haward, in a series of double-blind studies with normal volunteers, demonstrated that PHT improved cog-nitive function. In the United States, perhaps the most significant of these early studies was by Stephens and Shaffer at Johns Hopkins. In a double-blind crossover study, they found PHT to be markedly effective in reduc-ing symptoms related to fear and anger.

During this period Dr. Turner was searching the med-ical literature to see if previous work had been done on PHT. To my surprise he and his staff found hundreds of studies, published over the previous twenty years. These studies, in addition to confirming our observations in thought and mood, reported PHT to be useful for a variety of other disorders. Among them were cardiac disorders, trigeminal neuralgia, migraine, diabetes, pruritis ani, ulcers, and asthma.

* * *

Three years after I had met with Secretary Gardner, I was ready to go back to the government. When I had seen the Secretary I didn't have a lot of evidence. But now I was loaded for bear. This was a mistake. I should have brought an elephant gun. Republicans were in.

In the sequence of events we come to President Richard M. Nixon. By chance I knew Mr. Nixon before he became President. I'd seen his interview on "The David Susskind Show," and as a result, without being asked, had contributed to his presidential campaign. When Mr. Nixon was defeated I got to know him. When he lost the race for Governor of California I knew he had no chance to become President. If you can't win your own state, you can't win the United States.

That's what I thought, but Mr. Nixon was nominated for President in 1968. Again I contributed to his campaign; I also contributed to the campaign of Senator Hubert Humphrey. And I did what I suppose was an unusual thing. I told each I was contributing to the campaign of the other. In this matter of public health, it was important for me to be known by whichever one became President. I was able to talk to both before the election. With Mr. Nixon, I had a long conversation about PHT at Key Biscayne.

My discussion with Senator Humphrey about PHT took place at his headquarters in New York. When we finished he said, "Listen, son [that nearly got my vote], whether I win or lose, I want you to get back to me on this." I couldn't have hoped for anything nicer than that. After the election I was anxious to get back to the Senator but it took three months to get an appointment. We had coffee in his suite at the Waldorf-Astoria. He showed up from a bedroom in shirt sleeves, and I had the feeling we were going to get down to work. I started off enthusiastically. Then I noticed there was no response in his face, and his gaze was fixed on a picture on the wall in back of me. In about fifteen minutes my enthusiasm started to run down. When I left soon after, I had the feeling that Senator Humphrey was relieved. I was too, but deeply disappointed.

* * *

After Mr. Nixon became President I waited a few months for him to settle into position, so to speak, and then called Rose Mary Woods, his nice and well-known secretary. I spoke to her for quite a while, explaining what an urgent medical matter this was, and told her I would send her some written information. I asked her to please not talk to the President about it, just give it some thought and advise me on the best way to approach him on the matter. I'm really dumber than the law allows. Of course Rose Mary, as any good secretary would, told President Nixon about it. A few days later she called to tell me the material had been sent to Secretary of Health Finch and I would hear from him shortly. I had hoped to see the President himself, but this was fine. I waited to hear from Secretary Finch.

Days went by without my hearing from the Secretary and I started to get restless. By the time three months had elapsed I was beside myself (not easy). I didn't have sense

enough, or guts enough, to pick up the phone and call
Secretary Finch, so I spoke to a friend who had a friend
who knew the Secretary. This worked. Apparently the material Miss Woods had sent three months earlier hadn't
reached Secretary Finch on the conveyor belt that carries
things to the desk of a Secretary of Health. I got a call from
Secretary Finch's secretary and an appointment was made.

Dr. Bogoch and I met with Secretary Finch in his office
in December 1969. The Secretary didn't say whether he
had discussed the matter with President Nixon, but he'd
had a chance to look at the material I had sent the President, the *Life* and *Reader's Digest* articles, excerpts from
letters from physicians, and a condensed version of the
Worcester Jail Study. I hadn't wanted to burden the President with medical studies. But for the Secretary of Health
I brought, in a bulging briefcase, hundreds of medical
studies on the use of PHT for a variety of disorders. The
Secretary was impressed.

After we'd been with Secretary Finch a short while, he
asked Dr. Jesse L. Steinfeld, who had been appointed Surgeon General the previous day, to join us. Then, with both
present, Dr. Bogoch and I briefly summarized the clinical
evidence and basic mechanisms of action of PHT.

When we finished I told Secretary Finch about my
meeting with Secretary Gardner three years earlier, and
the advice he'd given me. Since that time so much new
information had come into the possession of the Dreyfus
Medical Foundation, facts not generally known, there was
no question that this was now a matter for the government.
To convey the information to the government, Dr. Bogoch
and I proposed that we have a two-day conference with a
broadly representative group of government physicians,

including members of the FDA. At such a conference we would present the medical information, and the government would be able to take it from there.

After we had made our proposal, Secretary Finch turned to the Surgeon General and said, "Let's get moving on this. How long will it take you to get a group together to meet with the Dreyfus Medical Foundation? How soon can you get a conference set up?"

"Probably in a couple of weeks," Dr. Steinfeld said.

"Well, do it faster if you can, but do it within two weeks," Secretary Finch told him. Apparently my sense of urgency had been picked up by the Secretary. We thanked him, and after exchanging telephone numbers with Dr. Steinfeld, Dr. Bogoch and I left with the feeling that the government would soon play its part.

When we got back to New York, Dr. Bogoch and I started the hard work of getting the data organized for the conference in two weeks. Four days went by before it occurred to me that we hadn't heard from the Surgeon General. Although Secretary Finch had given him explicit instructions to hold this meeting without delay, I thought it possible Dr. Steinfeld might be waiting for a call from me. I phoned him. His secretary said he was in conference and would call back. He didn't call back and I called again the next day. He was still in conference. This was the beginning of my awareness that phoning the Surgeon General and getting to speak to him were not exactly the same thing.

Several days later the Surgeon General called to say that he had been thinking about the conference; he thought we should have a meeting to discuss it and would like to have Dr. Bert Brown, head of the National Institute

of Mental Health, with him. We were prepared to meet
without delay, but he said he would be tied up for a week
and suggested that the four of us meet in Washington on
January 14. I could see that things were not going as
smoothly as I'd hoped; the meeting to discuss the meeting
that was supposed to have taken place in two weeks,
wouldn't take place for three weeks.

On the fourteenth we arrived in Washington to have
dinner with Dr. Steinfeld and Bert Brown. Dr. Brown was
not present. The Surgeon General explained that his secretary had forgotten to invite him. Without Dr. Brown the
Surgeon General felt we didn't have a "quorum" and
would have to have another meeting. We were taken
aback. Still, we felt the time could be put to good use if we
enlarged on Dr. Steinfeld's sketchy background on PHT.
We did our best, but we didn't seem to have the Surgeon
General's full attention because he would frequently in-
terject, "I don't know how my secretary forgot to call Dr.
Brown."

Before we left Washington we discussed our next
meeting with Dr. Steinfeld. Where we should meet
seemed a problem to him. He said maybe we should meet
in a motel. I didn't know what that meant, but to get things
moving I would have met in the men's room. We left
Washington with no definite date. I began to have the feeling that I was looking at the "Finch medical conference"
through the wrong end of a telescope.

I was not born with an oversupply of patience. Even
with Dilantin I am short of perfection. This is to explain to
the reader that the next six months were about as frustrating and exasperating a period of time as one could hope
not to enjoy. It was that long before we had another meet-

ing with the Surgeon General, this time with Dr. Brown. Both before and after this meeting, with a skill unequalled in my experience, Jesse ducked and dodged, retreated and sidestepped, and left me so off balance that I felt something was going to happen any day. Each time I managed to catch the Surgeon General on the telephone, a new subject would come up for consideration, such as, what physicians we should bring with us, where the meeting should take place, how many people should attend, what medical disciplines should be represented, and who should chair the meeting. (It was finally decided that Jesse should chair it.) It could have been chaired by Little Orphan Annie because the meeting never took place.

We kept contact with the Surgeon General, and this mirage of a meeting, for well over a year. His superb talent for keeping our interest alive, without doing anything other than that, explains why we did not think of going back to Secretary Finch until it was too late. (He left office six months after we met.)

The end came in the following way. We had gotten the Surgeon General pinned down to a meeting, the date made well in advance and its importance emphasized. Dr. Bogoch and I were going to review the medical data at length, feeling that this would motivate Dr. Steinfeld to set up the conference without further delay. And I was determined at this meeting to lay it on the line—either get results, or not.

A few days before the scheduled meeting I got a telephone call from Dr. Steinfeld's secretary saying she was sorry but we'd have to cancel the meeting for the coming Monday. I said, "But we had things all arranged for a full presentation. Why can't he make it?"

"He has to go out West on Monday to investigate the earthquake," she said. (An earthquake had occurred in California a week earlier.) If Jesse had been going to California to prevent the earthquake, well, good luck. But to cancel a medical meeting of this importance to visit an earthquake that had already happened, and not even propose a new date for the meeting, was too much. I said to myself, The heck with it, and Jesse didn't have any more of my phone calls to dodge.

I never did find out what a Surgeon General was supposed to do. He didn't do surgery, and he didn't command troops. Maybe the government couldn't find out either because when Dr. Steinfeld left, the office was retired.*

At the time Dr. Steinfeld left government, *The New York Times* reported him to have said that Federal health affairs were in a "kind of chaos." He was "frustrated seeing how much good I might have achieved and how much was actually accomplished."

In a nutshell.

* * *

I had placed a lot of hope on the government's taking over PHT. I admit that part of this was because I wanted to be relieved of the responsibility and the work. But there was a more important reason. With its medical institutions, and its enormous resources and authority, the government could do a far better job than a single foundation. However, it wasn't long after the Finch conference that I began to get the idea that government lacked enthusiasm about taking over its responsibilities.

---

* The office of Surgeon General has been resurrected. We wish the new Surgeon General, Dr. C. Everett Koop, the best of luck.

Maybe I should sum up my thoughts during this period. At the outset, when I became convinced that PHT had been overlooked, I knew that medical studies would be necessary to persuade others. After the initial unsuccessful attempts, the Foundation had sponsored numerous successful studies on PHT and was continuing in this effort. But by far the most important source of evidence was already in the medical literature. This evidence had been there for the picking, like good apples under a tree.

I don't know exactly when we passed the equator of ample evidence, but at some point our goal changed, and we decided that communicating already existing evidence was more important than finding new evidence. You know that old philosophical question about the tree falling in the forest—if nobody hears it, was there a sound? I'm not sure about that, but here was a practical question. If a great amount of evidence exists for the usefulness of a medicine, and the physician doesn't know about it, does it do any good? The answer is obvious. So communication became our number one objective.

Something other than trying to tell the story to the government had to be done. By this time we had collected so many published studies on PHT they would have filled a barrel. I would like to have Xeroxed the studies and sent each physician a barrelful saying, "You'll find this useful." But it wasn't practical. We had to attack the barrel ourselves, organize the studies, and condense them for the physicians. And that is what we did.

When we finished we had a bibliography and review of PHT, the clinical section arranged chronologically, the contents fairly evenly divided between clinical and basic mechanism of action studies. It was exhausting work for our group, and just the writing of it took over a year and a half. To keep our spirits up we worked on the theory that if a doctor matched a thousand hours of our effort with ten minutes of his own (aye, there's the rub) we'd show a profit —with 350,000 doctors in the U.S.A. The bibliography, *The Broad Range of Use of Phenytoin,* was the first of two that the Foundation published. About 400,000 copies were sent to physicians and basic scientists in the United States in 1970. The response was excellent, and we had letters of thanks from nearly a thousand physicians. Still, the facts about PHT did not spread as fast as I had hoped.

* * *

One Sunday morning in July 1971, my brain was playing with the communication problem. The Foundation was sponsoring studies of PHT, mostly in new fields, but we had no other immediate plans. The thought that government had the key responsibility for PHT was always in my mind. But I had taken my best shot with the government—President, Secretary of Health, and Surgeon General. Something else had to be done; I couldn't figure out what, and it bugged me.

It's funny how we remember unimportant things if they are associated with something important. That Sunday, my housekeeper Ida Thomas, whom I love and who has a feeling for me, sensed my mood and said, "Let me fix you something for breakfast instead of those old eggs and tomatoes you eat every day." I thanked her, and went back to thinking about the government. Interesting smells started coming out of the kitchen. Soon a delicious-looking pancake arrived, with powdered sugar and hot blueberry sauce. The first bite was on my fork when the phone rang.

A voice said, "This is Walter Tkach at the White House. I'm President Nixon's doctor, and I was just telling the President and Mrs. Nixon what a wonderful piece of work I thought you'd done." If an ancestor had called I couldn't have been more surprised. Just when I was wondering how to get back to the government, here was a spontaneous recommendation to the President, from his own doctor. I steadied my voice and thanked Dr. Tkach. Dr. Tkach went on to say, "The President suggested that I invite you to visit me in Washington and I hope you can make it soon." I said I could. We made a date for the following Tuesday. Then I ate Ida's pancake—and two more.

Tuesday I took a sensible morning plane to Washington that got me there at a quarter-to-ten. Dr. Tkach met me and drove me to the White House in his car. During the drive he told me that after a personal loss he'd benefited from PHT, and had the *Life* article to thank for it. I was glad he had firsthand experience with PHT; there's nothing like it to get an understanding of the medicine.

When we got to the White House, Dr. Tkach walked me past the gendarmes, and for a moment I had the feeling I was infiltrating the place. But when we got to his office Walter made me feel like a dignitary. He put me in a comfortable chair, got me a jug of coffee, and became a voluntary and patient listener for several hours. In that sympathetic atmosphere I did a good job of summarizing the PHT story.

At about twelve-thirty Dr. Tkach suggested lunch would be appropriate. He didn't have to drag me; I've always noticed that mental effort uses more calories than physical effort, and we went to the White House cafeteria. Walter hadn't told me we would have company for lunch, but he had invited Kenneth R. Cole, Jr., and James H. Cavanaugh, two members of the President's staff, to join us. I didn't get to eat as well as I'd hoped because I had to give a forty-five-minute summary of PHT. I emphasized the government's responsibility. Ken and Jim ate well and listened well.

When lunch was over Ken Cole, who outranked Jim Cavanaugh on the President's staff, said they would both try to be helpful in getting the story to the FDA. He said I could call him whenever necessary, but Jim would work with me on a regular basis. In the past I had been treated with courtesy by the government, but I'd felt a little like a salesman, carrying samples in his briefcase. Now I was being offered help without soliciting it and it put me in a different posture. When lunch was over I thanked them all.

Dr. Tkach drove me back to the airport. He said there wasn't any question that the government should do something about the PHT matter. But he cautioned me against being too optimistic. He said the problem wouldn't be with people I would meet but with the nature of bureaucracy. It was so big, and so besieged on all sides by people clamoring for its attention, that it was distracted from important matters—even if it could figure out which they were. A few years earlier I would have argued with Walter. Now I just kept my fingers crossed.

That same week Jim Cavanaugh came to New York and spent a day with Dr. Bogoch and me. It was one of those calorie-consuming days. I spent at least four hours going over clinical evidence, and Sam spent nearly half that time on the basic mechanisms. When he left, Jim had a good grasp of the facts. He said the next move would be for us

to talk to Dr. Charles Edwards, Commissioner of the FDA.
Jim Cavanaugh made the appointment with Commissioner Edwards, and Dr. Bogoch and I spent a morning in the offices of the FDA. After a long talk with the Commissioner, he said he'd like us to explain this matter to senior members of his staff. I don't remember their names, I saw them only once, but they were sympathetic and tried to be helpful. After we outlined the story, they told us that the Foundation itself might be able to apply for new listings of PHT. They suggested that Dr. Herbert Ley, the previous Commissioner of the FDA, would be a good person to consult about procedure.* I didn't understand why the Foundation should apply to the FDA in a matter of health for the American public when that health was a direct responsibility of the FDA itself.

Still, I would have considered following the suggestion except for two reasons. One was that PHT appeared to be useful for so many disorders that to get them through the FDA in the routine way, single file so to speak, would have taken forever. The second reason was that if the Foundation did make applications for new uses of PHT, we might be required to be silent on the subject while applications were pending. We couldn't risk that.

Dr. Edwards visited the Foundation a few weeks later. When he had spent most of a day absorbing the medical information, he agreed that a conference with medical officials would be appropriate and said he would help set up such a conference.

* We got in touch with Dr. Herbert Ley. Dr. Ley said he would like to review the summaries of the PHT studies in our bibliography; they seemed almost too good to be true. After spot-checking the summaries for a long day he was satisfied. Since then, Dr. Ley has been a consultant for the Foundation.

Dr. Edwards made the arrangements and a two-day conference was held in our offices in February 1972. Since Dr. Edwards had already spent a day with us on PHT, he attended only the first day of the meeting. Others in attendance were Dr. Theodore Cooper (Director, the National Heart and Lung Institute), Dr. John Jennings, Dr. James Pittman, Dr. Samuel Kaim, James Cavanaugh, Dr. Samuel Bogoch, and myself.

This conference was hard work. There were four two-hour sessions in the two days. Dr. Bogoch and I conducted them and, except during the discussion periods, we did all the talking. I assure you I looked forward to lunch and coffee breaks (see Agenda, p. 91–92).

By the time we got to the last discussion period, on the afternoon of the second day, the clinical effects of PHT and its basic mechanisms of action had been outlined, and we got down to cases—what the government could do. But none of our visitors could think of a handle for the FDA to grab PHT by; nothing like this had happened before. The only suggestion I remember was that perhaps the government could give the Foundation a grant. I appreciated this, but I didn't want us to lose any freedom of action.

As the meeting was breaking up, Dr. Kaim said to me, "Well, the ball is in your court." This struck my unfunny bone. "In my court?" I said. "Where the devil do you think it's been all these years—and when should it get in your court?" As many of us do, I make the mistake of thinking that an individual in the government is the government itself. Dr. Kaim meant no harm by his comment, but I repeat it because it is typical of a thousand I've heard from people in a position to do something about PHT themselves. They seem to clear their consciences by giving me advice as to what I should do. I've got enough of this

DREYFUS MEDICAL FOUNDATION
CONFERENCE ON PHT WITH FDA
February 22 and 23, 1972

Tuesday, February 22

10:00 A.M.   Background
Early evidence
Institutional studies (with reference to both crime
and problems within the institutions):
Worcester County Jail Study (double-blind)
Lyman School for Boys (Juvenile Delinquents)
Patuxent Institution

1:00 P.M.   Lunch

2:00 P.M.   Basic mechanisms of action of PHT:
Effect on hyperexcitable nerve cell
Suppression of post-tetanic potentiation
Stabilization of membrane
Regulatory effect on sodium and potassium
Resistance to anoxia
Increase of energy compounds in brain
(glucose, ATP, and creatine phosphate)
Stabilizing effects on labile diabetes
Cerebral and coronary vessel dilatation
Protection against digitalis toxicity
Protection against cortisone toxicity
Other anti-toxic effects of interest: DDT,
cyanide, alloxan, radiation, etc.

3:15 P.M.   Coffee and Discussion

3:30 P.M.   "The Broad Range of Use of PHT"
Review of thought, mood, and behavior disorders
(1938–1971)
Discussion

5:00 P.M.   Recess

7:30 P.M.   Dinner

Wednesday, February 23

9:00 A.M.   Review of "The Broad Range of Use of PHT"

(continued)

	Symptoms and disorders for which PHT effectiveness has been reported
	Discussion of cardiac uses
	Brief review of other somatic disorders
	Alcoholism and drug addiction
	Safety and toxicology
10:15 A.M.	Coffee
10:30 A.M.	The effects of PHT on overthinking, anger, fear, and related emotions
	The One-Hour test
11:30 A.M.	Recent work reporting therapeutic benefits of PHT in glaucoma, steroid myopathy, hostility in chronic psychotics, violence, radiation, shock lung, asthma, digitalis toxicity, and hypertension
12:30 P.M.	Lunch
1:30 P.M.	PHT's value is based on the combination of many factors:
	Broad range of effectiveness
	Rapidity of action
	Beneficial "side effects"
	Not addictive
	Not a sedative at therapeutic doses
	Safety established by long period of use
	How PHT has been overlooked
	Discussion
4:00 P.M.	Conference ends

advice. It's saved up in a hermetically sealed tank and I plan to sell to a utility—when fuel prices rise a bit more.

Although nothing specific came of the meeting, at least some members of the government had a better understanding of PHT. Jim Cavanaugh kept in touch with me regularly. Jim had a way of saying, "I'll get back to you next week." And he always did. I appreciated his efforts so much that I never pressed him as to when he would call. It was usually about a quarter to five—on Friday.

Occasionally I was able to get Commissioner Edwards on the phone. Charlie, who told me he was trying to work out something with members of the department, finally came up with a suggestion. He said that if we could get a political figure to write a letter of inquiry about PHT to Secretary of Health Richardson, the reply—which would be an official statement and could be made public—might shed light on the matter. By that time I was so worn out I would have settled for an old shoe. But Dr. Edwards' idea seemed constructive.

Since the Foundation was located in New York, I asked Dr. Edwards if a letter from Governor Rockefeller would serve the purpose. He said it would. When I asked Governor Rockefeller, to whom I had spoken previously about PHT, he said he would write such a letter. And he did.

Secretary Richardson's response* meant more to me than it would to someone unfamiliar with the background.

* From Secretary Richardson's letter:
"Conversations with health officials within the Department have revealed that phenytoin (PHT) was introduced in 1938 as the first essentially nonsedating anticonvulsant drug . . .

"A review of the literature reveals that phenytoin has been reported to be useful in a wide range of disorders. Among its reported therapeutic actions are its stabilizing effect on the nervous system, its antiarrhythmic effect on certain cardiac disorders, and its therapeutic effect on emotional disorders.

"The fact that such broad therapeutic effects have been reported by many independent scientists and physicians over a long period of time would seem to indicate that the therapeutic effects of phenytoin are more than that of an anticonvulsant.

"The FDA encourages the submission of formal applications. . . ."

(For the full text, see Appendix, p. 163.)

It showed that the Foundation's efforts had had some effect. The Secretary's comment, "Conversations with health officials in the Department . . ." indicated the letter had FDA approval.

* * *

I invaded the U.S. Government only once more. About two months into President Nixon's second term, I made one more try. I called Rose Mary Woods and told her the PHT matter was just too important to hang in limbo any longer. I had done the best I could with government for the last four years and now I needed Presidential advice. Rose Mary understood, and a few days later called back to say a date had been set up for lunch with the President—I should come at eleven-thirty so we would have more time to talk about PHT. Perfect.

I couldn't be late for such an appointment and planned to go to Washington the day before. But when I found the chance for rain approached zero, I made a reservation for a flight scheduled to get to Washington at nine-fifteen, which gave me almost two hours leeway. That darn plane ("Doing What We Do Best") managed to be two-and-a-half hours late and I was thirty-five minutes late for my appointment. If that wasn't embarrassing. But no one other than myself appeared ruffled. The President set me at ease and listened closely to my experiences with the government. I told him the situation was incredible. Everyone had tried to be helpful, but they were so busy with problems they didn't have time for a solution. I said I couldn't get it out of my head that if someone with authority had the facts he'd see to it that something got done in this matter so urgent to public health.

The PHT story was not new to the President, having heard it from me on three occasions. He agreed that something should be done and asked for my suggestion. I had anticipated the possibility that he might ask. I told him that political jokes for at least a century suggested that vice-presidents of the United States were not overworked. I said that if this applied to Vice-President Agnew, he might be able to help. This suggestion got a prompt Presidential veto (I lacked the two-thirds majority to overrule).

The President said he thought Secretary of Health Casper Weinberger would be the man for me to see. I told him I had already seen two Secretaries of HEW and found them pretty busy; on average I'd spent an hour apiece with them. This time I had to have enough time to tell the whole story. He asked how long this would take. I said at least two days, at a quiet place away from the telephone. I thought this was shooting for the moon, but the President saw the sense in it. He said he'd make arrangements, that at the moment the Secretary was up to his elbows in some matter, but I would hear from him within thirty days. I thanked the President and took a plane back to New York. Of course it got there two minutes early.

Back home I waited for Secretary Weinberger's call. After four weeks went by I began to have Finch flashbacks. But, on the twenty-ninth day, Secretary Weinberger called and made a date to spend the following weekend at Hobeau Farm. Mrs. Weinberger came to the farm with the Secretary and Dr. Bogoch was with me. Over the two days we had four long sessions, during which Dr. Bogoch and I poured information about PHT into the Secretary. Mrs. Weinberger was an interested listener.

Late Sunday we went our separate ways, the Weinbergers to Washington, Dr. Bogoch and I to New York. Caspar said he wanted to cogitate on the matter and would get in touch with me soon. Time went by, more than I'd expected, and I was afraid I had struck a black hole (a semi-anachronism—they were around in those days but who knew). But after two months Secretary Weinberger called and invited me to come to Washington to meet the newly appointed Commissioner of the FDA, Dr. Alexander Mackay Schmidt.

Our meeting was in the office of our friend, Charlie Edwards, who had become assistant head of HEW. Secretary Weinberger was present, but I got the feeling that, not being a physician, he was reluctant to make suggestions of a medical nature to the FDA, and he had asked Dr. Edwards, who knew the subject well, to introduce Dr. Bogoch and me to Dr. Schmidt.

After the introductions we all chatted for a few minutes in Dr. Edwards' office about nothing I can remember. Then Dr. Schmidt and Dr. Bogoch and I went off to another room to have a talk. I assumed, of course, that Dr. Edwards or the Secretary had given Dr. Schmidt the bibliography of the Dreyfus Medical Foundation and a thorough briefing on the nature of our interest in PHT. I was totally unprepared for Dr. Schmidt's opening words, "My number one objective in my new position is to see that the FDA is run in an honest and honorable fashion."

Son-of-a-gun!

After all the years of work with the government it was apparent Dr. Schmidt hadn't even been briefed. I was back at the starting line, with a new Commissioner of the FDA, and the baton hadn't even been passed on.

I considered getting up and going home. But I wasn't

delighted with the implications of Dr. Schmidt's opening remark, and I wanted to get that straightened out. I told Dr. Schmidt we were a charitable medical foundation, had no private interest of any sort, but a damned important public one, and that trying to be helpful with our government was getting to be a tiresome job.

Dr. Schmidt's response was a lot nicer than I expected. He said, "Take your time and tell me about it." For the umpteenth time I started telling the story of PHT.

After about an hour Dr. Schmidt said he had an appointment that he couldn't get out of, but he saw how important this was and he intended to pursue it personally. He said of course he knew PHT was more than an anticonvulsant. In fact he had been teaching its use in cardiac arrhythmia since 1969. I said that's just one example of what I'm talking about. "As you know, PHT does not have a listed indication-of-use for arrhythmias." Dr. Schmidt said, "You're mistaken. I'm sure PHT has such a listing." I didn't argue, this not being an opinion but a fact that could be checked. But I said I thought I was right.*

Just before we left, Dr. Schmidt mentioned that he was a specialist in communication. I said, "I've come to believe that communication is just a word in the dictionary, but if there is such a thing, you sure have a good spot to use your specialty."

Well, it turned out that Commissioner Schmidt was a

---

* A week later Dr. Schmidt called to say that it was hard to believe, but PHT did not have a listed indication-of-use for arrhythmias. The head of the Heart and Lung Institute, Dr. Theodore Cooper, had made the same mistake. At our medical conference, he had said, "There is no question of the usefulness of PHT as an antiarrhythmic, and this is an approved indication-of-use in the package insert."

That was years ago. PHT still doesn't have such a listing.

gentleman of the old school (an endangered species). Even with the pressures of his new office he kept his promise to look into PHT himself and visited the Foundation twice in the following month. The second time, he spent a full day getting the facts about PHT from Dr. Bogoch and me and even stayed into the evening so we could finish our discussion at dinner. By that time I had a feeling of empathy with Mack, and with the help of a glass of wine, I emptied myself of my feelings on the subject of the great sin of neglect of PHT. Dr. Schmidt understood. Then he said something I'd been hoping to hear from a government official but had given up on. "You've done what you can. Now the ball is in our court."

Well, that was it; there was no more to do. I had been trying to turn the responsibility for PHT over to the U.S. government for ten years. Finally a Commissioner of the FDA had accepted it.

* * *

Epilogue: Of course I should have figured that a man as sensitive as Mack Schmidt wouldn't last long in government. Five months later he was back at the University of Illinois, and there was a new Commissioner of the FDA.

I have not visited the government since and have no ambition to. That's one reason this book is written. It's for members of the staff and government officials in health, all at the same time. I hope it will make it easier for them to do whatever they think is right.

10.
TRAVELS ABROAD
England—Italy—Russia

It's said that the further you get from where they know you the more respect you get. And so it seems.

Before discussing the "flaw in the system," in the next chapter, I would like to tell you of some experiences I've had with PHT abroad, and of an unusual relationship that developed between the Dreyfus Medical Foundation and the Institute for Experimental Medicine in Leningrad.

England

My first trip abroad, on the subject of PHT, was to England in 1965. Soon after Dr. Turner joined the Foundation, he and I went to Chichester, England, to visit a friend of his, Dr. Lionel Haward. At the Graylingwell Hospital in Chichester, Dr. Haward introduced us to a group of his colleagues. We all sat at a large round table and for an hour I described my experiences with PHT. When I finished, to my surprise, they applauded. I know it was just English good manners but it gave me a nice feeling.

As a result of our trip, Dr. Haward did a series of five controlled studies on PHT.* They were excellent studies,

* See *The Broad Range of Clinical Use of PHT*, p. 11, 13–14.

three of them unusual in that they were influenced by his background as a pilot. In simulated air control tests, he demonstrated with students and experienced pilots that PHT was significantly effective in delaying fatigue and accompanying errors. Haward made the point that it's an unusual substance that can calm without sedation and also effect a return of energy and improvement in concentration.

Italy

Dr. Rodolfo Paoletti, scientific director of the Institute of Pharmacology at the University of Milan, a friend of Dr. Bogoch's, frequently visited our office when in New York. On several occasions I talked to him about PHT. One of the times Dr. Paoletti said, "Why don't you come over to Milan and talk about PHT at a meeting of the Giovanni Lorenzini Foundation." He suggested a date four months in the future and I accepted.

A week before the meeting I found out what I had let myself in for. I was not to be one of many speakers, but the only speaker, before a large group of physicians. I had talked at formal medical meetings before, but only as one of the speakers. This was different.

At the meeting in Milan there were about 120 physicians. Dr. Paoletti gave me a kind introduction, put me on the podium with a microphone attached to me, and told me to speak in my normal way—a UN-type device would see that it came out in Italian. I was close to stage fright, but after I got started it was all right. I talked for an hour and twenty minutes, and apparently it went well because

I got a letter from Dr. Paoletti saying, "From the comments I heard afterward you certainly caught everyone's attention," and he invited me to come back the next year.

After the meeting a number of physicians came up to say hello, and I learned that PHT was already being used for purposes other than epilepsy. One physician, G. A. Bozza, who seemed an especially kind man, talked to me about his use of PHT with retarded children, a use I was not familiar with. A few months later he sent me his paper, "Normalization of intellectual development in the slightly brain-damaged, retarded child."*

Russia

One day in October 1972, Dr. Bogoch phoned and said he was coming to the office with a Russian doctor he thought I'd like to meet, and that we might have lunch. The doctor was in New York for an International Brain Sciences Conference, of which Dr. Bogoch was chairman. At eleven o'clock that morning Dr. Bogoch arrived in the office with Dr. Natasha Bechtereva. Sam had not overdescribed Dr. Bechtereva when he referred to her as a Russian doctor. Dr. Bechtereva had the most impressive credentials of anyone I've met in the medical profession.

At that time Dr. Bechtereva was Chairman of the Commission on Public Health of the U.S.S.R. She was also Director (and still is) of the Institute for Experimental Medicine, formerly the Pavlov Institute, a group of seven large hospitals in Leningrad. Dr. Bechtereva was the first

* Presented at the Italian National Conference of Child Neuropsychology, 1971.

woman to become Director of the Institute and she was Chief of its neurophysiological branch.

I remember our meeting clearly. Dr. Bechtereva, Dr. Bogoch, and I sat in chairs at a window overlooking New York Harbor. I had intended to talk about PHT for half an hour or so and, if Dr. Bechtereva showed interest, give her a copy of *The Broad Range of Use of Phenytoin*. When lunch arrived at one o'clock I was surprised to find that I'd been talking for two hours. Dr. Bechtereva hadn't said a thing, but the patience with which she had listened and something in her remarkable eyes had kept me going.

When I had finished Dr. Bechtereva spoke for the first time. She said, "What you say seems too good to be true but it's not illogical, and I can find out to my own satisfaction. In our Institute we have sensitive electrical equipment that can test PHT. Would you be kind enough to send us a supply of your brand of phenytoin? If our tests should disagree with what you say I wouldn't want you to think it's because our brand is different from yours." That made sense, and I said we would send the Dilantin.

After many difficulties, Dilantin arrived in Leningrad. Several months later I received a letter from Dr. Bechtereva (mail in those days took about a month—now it's not so rapid). Dr. Bechtereva's electrical instruments had not been disappointed. From the letter:

Thank you very much for the prospect of Dilantin and the Dilantin itself. The Dilantin—really a most peculiar medicine.

I am advising it to more and more people. I simply can't resist doing it—you know how one feels. And so, step by step, Dilantin is used for nonepileptic purposes, not only in Leningrad but in Moscow and Kiev as well.

Dr. Bechtereva has a refreshing way of putting things. In a later letter she said, "People use Dilantin much more, though it met the normal prejudice determined by the engram fixed in each doctor's memory: Dilantin → epilepsy." Apparently we don't have a monopoly on this engram.

A few months after Dr. Bechtereva started work with PHT, she invited Dr. Bogoch and me to visit the Institute in Leningrad, at our convenience. We accepted. Having heard too much about the Russian winters we selected June for the visit. Four of us made the trip—Dr. Bogoch and his wife Dr. Elenore Bogoch, and Joan Personette, my former wife, and I.

We stayed in Leningrad for a week at the Hotel Astoria, a very old hotel, like the Ritz in Paris, but otherwise dissimilar. But the people were nice, which is the most important thing. When we had time we saw the sights, the beautiful cathedrals and the extraordinary Hermitage, and we walked around Leningrad as we pleased. The days were long. We were near the land of the midnight sun, and it got dark at 11 P.M. and light at 2 A.M. It seemed strange reading by daylight at 10 P.M. in a park across from the Astoria.

Dr. Bechtereva's hospitality was reminiscent of our best Southern hospitality. We had a delicious dinner at her home with her family, were taken out to dinner by her, and thoughtfully left to ourselves. The food in the restaurants was good, if you like garlic, which I don't. On one occasion, out to dinner with Dr. Bechtereva, I was trying to finesse my way around the meat and Natasha said, "My dear Jack, you suffer so much." A keen observer.

The first day we were in Leningrad, Dr. Bechtereva took the Drs. Bogoch and me to one of the seven hospitals and introduced us to key members of her staff. Later we went through other hospitals, getting to meet many doctors. I was surprised that so many of the doctors were women until I was told that seventy percent of physicians in Russia are women.

The second day we were there, Dr. Bechtereva introduced us to three patients who'd had dramatic benefits from PHT. Each had a different disorder. The patient I remember best was a woman who'd had severe headaches for many years and had to be hospitalized periodically. This time she had taken Dilantin for a few days and was on her way home. She explained, through an interpreter, that the pain in her head would get so bad she'd sit absolutely still and if anyone came near her it would make her furious. While she was explaining this in Russian, she was smiling happily, as though she were talking about someone else.

The next day Dr. Bechtereva called a meeting and Dr. Bogoch and I had the opportunity to talk about PHT to eighty physicians. I talked for about two hours. That was like talking one hour because translation was not simultaneous. Then Dr. Bogoch discussed the basic mechanisms of action. Several of the Institute's physicians also addressed the group. I was told that they had given favorable reports on PHT.

The day before we left, Dr. Bechtereva and I were alone for a few moments and I brought up what I considered a delicate subject. I told her that I was most impressed with the work the Institute had done. I said our Foundation had funded numerous studies on PHT, some outside the U.S.A., and, if proper, we would be happy to do it here. Natasha set me at ease. She said she appreciated my asking but that her Institute was well financed by the government. However, we might consider a "joint cooperative effort." She said such a possibility was provided for in the recent meeting between President Nixon and Premier Brezhnev.

I thought this a fine idea and asked how we should proceed. Dr. Bechtereva said since we had introduced the PHT idea it would be best if we initiated the matter through our Department of Health—to their Ministry of Health. We discussed it. Our thought was that we'd exchange ideas and information by mail, and would periodically visit each other. It was agreed that when I got back to New York I would introduce the matter to our Department of Health.

I won't bore you with details. The mills of government grind slowly all over the world. But in 1976, a formal approval was given for a "joint cooperative effort" between the Institute for Experimental Medicine and the Dreyfus Medical Foundation. I have been told that this is the only venture of its sort between a Russian and an American institution.

Before closing I'd like to say that Natasha Bechtereva is one of the most remarkable persons I've ever met, and I thank her for her help.

11.
A FLAW
IN THE SYSTEM

Parke-Davis—the Physician—the FDA

A medicine can get overlooked for a million years—if no one discovers it. But can the benefits of a discovered medicine get overlooked for decades when thousands of studies have demonstrated its usefulness? The answer is it can.

We have a flaw in our system of bringing prescription medicines to the public. That there's a flaw is no surprise. We're human and all our systems have flaws. But this particular flaw should be explained. It has acted like a barrier between the American public and a great medicine.

* * *

From drug company, through FDA, to physician—that's the route a prescription medicine takes to get to the public. That's our system. It was not set up by anyone, it just evolved. But we're used to it; it has become custom. And as you know, custom can be like iron.

Years ago doctors concocted their own medicines—and leeches outsold aspirins. But for the last century the business of pharmaceuticals has been in the hands of the drug companies. Drug companies, formed for the purpose of making money for shareholders, are not charged with a responsibility to the public that is not consistent with making money. That is not to suggest that drug companies are not interested in public welfare—but they are not charged with a responsibility for it.

In 1938 the FDA was empowered to protect us against medical substances more dangerous than therapeutic. Since that time drug companies have been required to get approval as to the safety of a new chemical entity and, since 1962, approval as to its effectiveness. Although the neglect of a great drug can be far more deadly than the use of a bad one, correcting such neglect does not appear to be a function of the FDA.

When a drug company synthesizes a compound which it believes to be therapeutic, it's brought to the FDA. If the drug satisfies that agency's requirements, the company is awarded a "listed indication-of-use," which permits it to market the drug. Getting FDA approval is time-consuming and expensive; it has been estimated, on average, to take seven years and to cost $11 million. (In 1988, the estimate of cost is far greater.)

Drug companies patent their new compounds. Patents give the company exclusive rights for seventeen years. If the FDA approves a drug and it becomes popular, the drug company has a winner since the drug will sell at a high price for the life of the patent.* However, when the patent expires, competition enters the picture and the price of the drug drops dramatically. At that point there is more financial incentive for the drug company to look for a *new drug* to patent than to look for new uses of an old drug.

FDA approval is the second of the three steps in our

---

* This is reasonable; a drug that is a winner has to pay for the research that went into it, the expense of getting FDA approval, and for money spent on the many drugs that are not successful.

system. The third step is the introduction of the drug to the physician. This is a function of the drug company and is done through advertisements in trade journals and by visits of their salesmen to physicians.

That is the system—and physicians have come to depend on it. If a doctor doesn't hear from a drug company about new uses for an old medicine, the doctor infers there aren't such uses. This is a reasonable inference. But in the case of PHT it's wrong.

So this is the flaw in the system. When a drug company doesn't do what is expected of it, and the FDA can't or doesn't do anything about it, the physician doesn't get vital information. And, as in this case, a great drug can get overlooked.

Parke-Davis

Parke-Davis's research did not discover PHT. The company bought the compound from a chemist in 1909. For twenty-nine years this remarkable drug sat on the shelf doing nobody any good. Then Putnam and Merritt, two physicians outside the company, discovered its first therapeutic use. Parke-Davis paid almost nothing in money for PHT. They paid less in brains for PHT.

Still, were it not for Parke-Davis we might not have PHT today. Someone in the company did buy the compound, and someone else in the company did give it to Putnam and Merritt for trial. It should also be said, to their credit, that Parke-Davis has been consistent in manufacturing a good product.

*   *   *

It is not easy to understand how a drug company can overlook its own product. An outline of my own experience with Parke-Davis may help.

In 1966, as Secretary Gardner had recommended, I made contact with Parke-Davis. I phoned the company and spoke to the president, Mr. H. W. Burrows. I told him of Secretary Gardner's recommendation that I speak to Parke-Davis, and supposed that would arouse his interest. But as I talked I didn't hear the noises one expects from an interested listener. To get his attention I said, "Look, I've spent $400,000 on your medicine and I don't want anything for myself, I just want to tell Parke-Davis about it." That got Mr. Burrows' attention. He said, "I wouldn't know anything about this, I'm just a bookkeeper."

That startling statement was my introduction to Parke-Davis. President Burrows said he would have someone get in touch with me. Two months later I got a call from Dr. Leon Sweet of Parke-Davis's research department. He was calling at Mr. Burrows' suggestion and made a date to meet with me in New York.

We met at my home. Dr. Sweet brought Dr. E. C. Vonder Heide with him. Dr. Turner was with me. Dr. Sweet said that Parke-Davis's recent head of research, Dr. Alain Sanseigne, had left the company a few months earlier to go to Squibb, and Dr. Vonder Heide, a former head of research now retired, had come along to be helpful.

Dr. Turner and I talked at length about the overlooked uses of PHT. Dr. Vonder Heide said it didn't surprise him that PHT was more than an anticonvulsant. In fact Parke-Davis had had numerous reports that Dilantin helped with alcohol and drug addiction. He said that he had tried to get doctors to conduct studies in this field without success. He was rather critical of the doctors. I remember thinking, What's going on here? The doctors depend on Parke-Davis to do something, and Parke-Davis depends on the doctors to do something. This is an interesting game of tag, and the public is "it."

I didn't realize till years later what a poor excuse Dr. Vonder Heide had given. Many research-minded doctors had already done a great deal, and at that time, 1966, Parke-Davis's files were stocked with a variety of clinical studies on PHT. Yet apparently neither Dr. Vonder Heide nor Dr. Sweet had heard of them. It seemed Parke-Davis's research department and its filing department were not acquainted with each other.

Our next contact with Parke-Davis came a few weeks later when we had a visit from a friendly gentleman, Dr. Charles F. Weiss. Dr. Weiss explained that he was a pediatrician and didn't know anything about PHT, but had come to see us because he'd been asked to. He offered the opinion that Parke-Davis was a little disorganized. He said he wished some company would take them over. Well, he got his wish—but not for six years. Today the company is a subsidiary of Warner Lambert.

When Warner Lambert took over in 1971, Mr. J. D. Williams became President of the Parke-Davis division. I felt I should bring the matter of PHT to the attention of the new management, and had several discussions on the telephone with Mr. Williams. The talks were friendly but not useful in furthering the PHT cause. On one occasion Mr. Williams expressed a thought I'd heard from Parke-Davis before, that since we were working on their product, it might be better if we stayed apart—some notion that the

FDA might like it better. I couldn't understand this—I was sure the FDA would want a drug company to know all it could about its own product.

But such is life. An item in the *Arizona Republic* (at the time I retired from Wall Street in 1970) will give the picture. The paper reported Dr. Joseph Sadusk, Vice-President for Medical and Scientific Research of Parke-Davis, to have said that the Dreyfus Medical Foundation is doing "an excellent job" in investigating PHT. As a result he said Parke-Davis has made only "a minimal effort" in this area of research. "Results from an unbiased third party like Dreyfus," he said, "would mean more to the Food and Drug Administration."

I appreciate compliments. But the division of labor seemed uneven. The Dreyfus Medical Foundation should do the research, influence the FDA—and Parke-Davis should make the profits.

There appears to have been only one person who, while passing through Parke-Davis, got a good grasp of PHT. That was Dr. Alain Sanseigne, head of research before Dr. Sweet. Dr. Turner brought PHT to Dr. Sanseigne's attention. Dr. Sanseigne graciously acknowledged this in a letter to Dr. Turner in which he said, "Your very thorough knowledge of Dilantin put me to shame."

Once his attention had been directed to PHT, Dr. Sanseigne, in 1965, reviewed its pharmacology, site of activity, and therapeutic activity.* It's an impressive review, and it

---

* From Dr. Sanseigne's review:
  The Parke-Davis Medical Brochure includes as indications of Dilantin the following:

Epilepsy	Migraine
Chorea	Trigeminal neuralgia
Parkinson syndrome	Psychosis

(*continued*)

refers only to information on PHT available over twenty years ago. There are no signs that this review stirred Parke-Davis.

When Dr. Joseph Sadusk said Parke-Davis's efforts had been "minimal" he selected the right word. I know this from firsthand experience. A few years ago Mr. Williams changed his mind about Parke-Davis staying apart from our Foundation and graciously arranged for three members of the research staff to meet with us on the subject of Parke-Davis's Dilantin package insert. (This package insert will be discussed later.)

At this meeting, I met the senior research officer of Parke-Davis. When we finished our discussion he mentioned that the FDA had not approved Parke-Davis's application for the use of PHT in cardiac arrhythmias. The reason, he said, was that the company did not supply cardiograms requested by an individual in the FDA. The research officer said, "We could get them for $100,000 but

---

The following indications . . . have been studied and seem to show considerable therapeutic response to treatment with PHT:

Cardiac arrhythmia	Wound-healing acceleration
Neurosis	Polyneuritis of pregnancy
Behavioral disorders	Tabetic lancinating pain
in adolescents	Pruritus ani
Myotonia	Asthma
Diabetes insipidus	

The following are indications on which the possibility of favorable response to PHT should be investigated:

Prophylaxis and treatment of	Wilson's disease
cerebral anoxia (carbon	Poorly controlled diabetes
monoxide poisoning and	Cicatrization of oral surgery
other asphyxiation, precardiac	Osteogenesis imperfecta
and pulmonary	Conditions related to hypo-
surgery)	thalamus

why spend the money, all the cardiologists are using PHT anyway." I won't take sides in this hassle between the FDA and Parke-Davis. There was foolishness to spare.* But you'd think Parke-Davis would have considered it a privilege to spend the $100,000.

A few weeks after this, a physician applied to our Foundation for a modest grant ($6,000). He had done interesting preliminary work on the use of PHT as a protection against brain damage after cardiac arrest. We intended to make the grant, but it occurred to me that the new Parke-Davis management might appreciate the opportunity. I called my new acquaintance, the research officer, and asked him about it. It didn't surprise me that I was told no. It did surprise me how quickly I got the answer, on the phone, without consideration of the matter. The senior officer explained that Parke-Davis was spending its research moneys on a new medicine the company hoped to patent. I thought there will be snow on the Devil's roof before they came up with as good a medicine as Dilantin. But I got the point—patents on PHT had expired.

Well, to sum up, Parke-Davis got Dilantin by luck. They didn't understand their own product, have done little to try to understand it, and haven't spent a bean in furthering its understanding. This has contributed to the overlooking of PHT.

But let's see Parke-Davis in perspective. There's no Mr. Parke, no Mr. Davis—just an entity with those names. Since Parke-Davis did not get PHT by the sweat of its research there was none of the interest in the drug that would be found in a company that developed its own prod-

* PHT is so widely used for cardiac arrhythmias that AMA Drug Evaluations has it in the category of antiarrhythmic agents.

uct. As a result, new uses for PHT was a job never assigned to anyone—and no one took it upon himself. It has been easy to cuss Parke-Davis, the entity, but not the people. In fact I've never met anyone at the company I didn't like.

* * *

About Parke-Davis's Dilantin package insert.

I was weaned on the Securities Exchange Commission. The S.E.C. is a fiend for full disclosure—the positive as well as the negative. If Parke-Davis operated under S.E.C. regulations the S.E.C. would have the company in court for the rest of the century because of the great amount of positive data that's not disclosed in their package insert.

But Parke-Davis operates under FDA regulations. Apparently full disclosure is required on the negative side, but no disclosure is permitted when the evidence is positive, unless it has an FDA listed indication-of-use. No matter how flimsy the evidence for the negative, it must be disclosed. No matter how solid the positive evidence, it may not be mentioned. It seems a poor way to run a railroad.

An example of inexplicable illogic. For some years prior to 1972, Parke-Davis's package insert made reference to a number of the uses of PHT other than epilepsy. In 1971 the insert stated: "Dilantin is also useful in the treatment of conditions such as chorea and Parkinson's syndrome and is employed in the treatment of migraine, trigeminal neuralgia and certain psychoses." In 1972 reference to these uses was deleted, although the evidence for their use had been substantially increased.

Unfathomable. I don't know whether this was the fault

of Parke-Davis or the FDA. But an innocent public has
suffered.

The Physician

A physician's remedy of the eighteenth century—from
A Majestic Literary Fossil by Mark Twain.

> **Aqua Limacum.** Take a great Peck of Garden-snails, and
> wash them in a great deal of Beer, and make your Chim-
> ney very clean, and set a Bushel of Charcoal on Fire; and
> when they are thoroughly kindled, make a Hole in the
> Middle of the Fire, and put the Snails in, and scatter
> more Fire amongst them, and let them roast till they
> make a Noise; then take them out, and, with a Knife and
> coarse Cloth, pick and wipe away all the green froth:
> Then break them, Shells and all, in a Stone Mortar. Take
> also a Quart of Earthworms, and scour them with Salt,
> divers times over. Then take two Handfuls of Angelica
> and lay them in the Bottom of the Still; next lay two
> Handfuls of Celandine; next a Quart of Rosemary-flow-
> ers; then two Handfuls of Bearsfoot and Agrimony; then
> Fenugreek, then Turmerick; of each one Ounce: Red
> Dock-root, Bark of Barberry-trees, Wood-sorrel, Betony,
> of each two Handfuls.—Then lay the Snails and Worms
> on top of the Herbs; and then two Handfuls of Goose
> Dung, and two Handfuls of Sheep Dung. Then put in
> three Gallons of Strong Ale, and place the pot where you
> mean to set Fire under it: Let it stand all Night, or
> longer; in the Morning put in three ounces of Cloves
> well beaten, and a small Quantity of Saffron, dry'd to
> Powder; then six Ounces of Shavings of Hartshorn,
> which must be uppermost. Fix on the Head and Refrig-
> eratory, and distil according to Art.

Serve with a shovel, no doubt.—Mark T.

I had taken PHT for about a year when I started talking to doctors about it. These were informal talks and occurred when chance brought me together with physicians, as at a dinner or in a locker room. I must have spoken to more than twenty doctors during that early period. None of them had heard of PHT being used for anything other than epilepsy. The discussions were friendly, but it was almost impossible to get a physician interested in the subject of PHT. I thought this was because, as a Wall Street man, I was an improbable source of medical fact.

But my lack of credentials was the smallest part of the communication problem. In the physicians' minds there was the fixed notion that PHT was just an anticonvulsant. They had been taught this in school, the "knowledge" had been in their heads for a long time, and had calcified. Don't pick on the physician. Calcification of ideas is a human trait not special to him.

There was an even bigger obstacle—the sure knowledge the physician had that if Dilantin had as many uses as I said it had, they would have heard about them from Parke-Davis. After all, Dilantin was their product, wasn't it? And they wanted to make money, didn't they? This "irrefutable logic" always defeated me. If I tried to explain, time would run out before we could get back to PHT.

There's been a recent trend to knock the doctor. I think it's a reaction to the pedestal position we had him in a decade ago. We learned from "Dr. Kildare" and "Marcus Welby, M.D." that there are two physicians to every patient. In real life this isn't so. Doctors rarely make house calls anymore. They can see three patients in the office for one in the home—and still it's hard to get an appointment.

Don't blame the doctor. It's the ecologists' fault—they've allowed the spread of *Homo sapiens* to get out of hand.

When you are giving a member of the medical profession a hard time (in your head of course—who would dare do it in person), consider that the doctor's day never ends. Sick people don't care what time it is, and the doctor has to go around with a beeper attached to him or be in constant touch with his telephone service. This means twenty-four hours' tension. We complain about what the doctor doesn't do. But do we appreciate the things he does that we wouldn't do?

*　*　*

We come to an important subject: medical literature. Medical studies are called literature (Shakespeare might demur) when they're published in a medical journal or as part of the record of a medical conference.

There is a great deal of this literature. You could wallpaper the world with it and have enough left over to do your kitchen. The notion that physicians know what's contained in the literature is bizarre. But some of them sound like they half believe they do. If you ask a physician a question he can't answer, don't be surprised if he responds, "Nobody knows." Which seems to suggest he has read all the literature and has total recall.

It's estimated that there are 3,300 medical journals in the world. A poll in seventeen counties of upstate New York (not exactly the boondocks) showed that the average physician subscribed to 4.1 of these journals. Double this figure if you like. Even if he read the 8.2 journals cover to cover, he would still be 3,291.8 journals short. You can see it's impossible to expect the physician to read the medical literature to determine which drugs he should use. That's why, in this day of specialization, this is left to the drug companies and the FDA.

However, when a physician gets a new idea about an established drug, he may apply it.* But the opportunity doesn't come up often. Usually new uses of a drug are well explored by the drug company that introduced it. PHT has been a marked exception, and a rare opportunity was presented to the physicians.

The medical profession did not fail us. The work of thousands of physicians has given us a rich literature on PHT. This literature, international in scope, covers a wide variety of medical disciplines. Published in many languages over a period of years, it is spread far and wide. But intermingled with millions of other studies, this literature is almost lost unless someone seeks it out.

The science fiction writer Robert Heinlein calls it the Crisis of the Librarian:

> The greatest crisis facing us is not Russia, not the Atom Bomb . . . It is a crisis in the *organization* and *accessibility* of human knowledge. We own an enormous "encyclopedia"—which isn't even arranged alphabetically. Our "file cards" are spilled on the floor, nor were they ever in order. The answers we want may be buried somewhere in the heap. . . .

Let me give you an example of how difficult it would be, even in a single field, for a physician to be acquainted

---

* Former FDA Commissioner Charles C. Edwards states: "Once the new drug is in a local pharmacy, the physician may, as part of the practice of medicine . . . vary the conditions of use from those approved in the package insert, without obtaining approval of the FDA." *The Federal Register, Vol. 37, No. 158, Aug. 15, 1972.* This was clearly restated in the April, 1982, *FDA Drug Bulletin.*

with the literature on PHT. Disorders in the field have many names. A general description of the field is uncontrolled muscle movement, or continuous muscle fiber activity.

To illustrate the point, we made up a table of twenty-one published studies on this subject in 1975.* These studies show dramatic recovery by patients given PHT. In many of the cases myogram readings (electrical muscle recordings) confirmed the clinical observations. The difficulty an individual physician would have in becoming acquainted with this work is shown by the following:

The studies were published in eight different countries, in sixteen different journals—Journal of Neurology, Neurosurgery and Psychiatry, Lancet, The Practitioner, South African Medical Journal, Klinische Wochenschrift, Arquivos de Neuro-Psiquiatria, Acta Neurologica, Proceedings of the Australian Association of Neurologists, Ceskolovenska Neurologie, Connecticut Medicine, Neurology, Archives of Neurology, New York State Journal of Medicine, California Medicine, and New England Journal of Medicine.

In only two of the twenty-one studies was the word phenytoin in the title. The other studies were published under such dissimilar titles that Scotland Yard couldn't have found them, without the key word phenytoin.

Some members of the medical profession have prescribed PHT for a variety of purposes for many years. The breadth of its use has been more than might be imagined. IMS America surveys the use of thousands of drugs. For

---

* Since then many more studies have been published, see *The Broad Range of Clinical Use of PHT*, p. 37–47.

their estimate of the many clinical conditions for which physicians are using PHT, see Appendix, p. 164–68.

One might draw the conclusion from the IMS America survey that the medical profession knows all about PHT. But this is not the case. Many physicians know of one or several uses of PHT. Few have an overall picture of the drug. Thus we have a strange situation. Dr. Jones prescribes PHT for depression. Dr. Smith uses it for migraine. Dr. Hemplewaith for trigeminal neuralgia. But, if a patient asks Dr. Snodgrass if he could try PHT for any of these purposes, he may get ushered from the office with the admonishment that PHT is only for epilepsy.

The right of a physician to prescribe whatever drug he wants is fundamental. But in making his decision he should have a reasonable amount of evidence on which to base his judgment. A reasonable amount of information has not been available to the physician, at least not from the expected source, the drug company. The information has been there, but it's been hidden in millions of medical papers, like trees in a forest.

When physicians know more about PHT they will realize they have been imposed on by the system—and deprived of a remarkable therapeutic tool.

The FDA

This is not going to be a treatise on the Food and Drug Administration. I haven't the facts or the desire to write such a treatise. The FDA is in this book because of its relation to PHT.

The FDA was established, in the best tradition of good government, to help American citizens in matters of health, in ways they can't help themselves. But it was conceived as a defensive unit. If it were a football team it would have six tackles and five guards, and no one to carry the ball. All that was expected of the FDA was defense— to protect us from dangerous substances and unwarranted claims of effectiveness.

Understandably the founding fathers of the FDA presumed that the drug companies, with their profit incentives, would furnish the offense. It could hardly have entered their minds that a drug company would leave a great medicine "lying around." Nor would they have been able to figure out how to equip the FDA against such an eventuality unless the FDA were put into the drug business, which is a far cry from the original premise—and is not being recommended here.

The FDA has done nothing about PHT. That is to be expected when a drug company doesn't play its role. Unfortunately this does not leave the FDA in a neutral position. Through no fault of the FDA's, PHT's narrow listing has a negative effect. Absence of FDA approval is thought of by many as FDA disapproval—or at the least that something is lacking. The system of drug company through FDA to physician has become such a routine that the physician, with other things on his mind, waits for the system to bring him PHT. It's been a long wait.

The real purpose in establishing the FDA was to improve the health and well-being of the citizens of the United States. The neglect of a great drug certainly falls into that category. If a man were drowning and a doctor was prepared to throw him a life preserver that had more lead than cork, the FDA would say, "Hold it! That thing might hit him and kill him, and even if it doesn't it can't help him." Nice work, FDA. But suppose the FDA knew there was a good life preserver under a tree, which the doctor didn't see. Shouldn't they say, "Try that one, Doc." Of course they should.

It is not suggested that the FDA go into the drug business. It is more than suggested, in this extraordinary case, where thousands of physicians have furnished us with many times the evidence required to get approval of a *new* drug (keep in mind this drug has been approved for comparative safety and has stood the test of over forty years of use), that the FDA should no longer take a hands-off policy. It's a sure thing our public shouldn't suffer any longer because Parke-Davis stayed in bed after Rip Van Winkle got up.

Let us understand the magnitude of what we're talking about. The non-use of PHT has been a catastrophe. We are not accustomed to thinking of the non-use of a medicine as a catastrophe. We think of a catastrophe as a flood, a famine, or an earthquake. Something tangible, overt, something in the positive tense. But something passive, such as the non-use of a great medicine that can prevent suffering and prolong lives, is also a catastrophe.

Something *must* be done. How it is done is for the government to decide. But here is a suggestion. It would seem a waste of time, and thus to the disadvantage of the American public, for the FDA to attempt to approve the many clinical uses of PHT separately. That could take forever. It would be far simpler for the FDA to address itself to the basic mechanisms of action and give PHT a listed indication-of-use as a stabilizer of bioelectrical activity, or as a membrane stabilizer. Certainly the published evidence for this is overwhelming. Such a listing would stimulate the physician to think of clinical applications of PHT and to refer to the existing medical literature.

Even a nod from the FDA to the physician would help. It could take the form of a letter to the physician, calling attention to the literature of his colleagues, and reminding him that since PHT has been approved for safety he is permitted to use it for whatever purposes his judgment suggests. Certainly the FDA would never try to tell the doctor how he should use PHT. That's always the doctor's decision. But such a letter would lift the cloud of negativism, and the physician would get an unobstructed view of PHT and the work of his colleagues.

I'm sure the problem agriculturists will say that if the FDA takes any action in this matter it will set a precedent. Fine. Good. If this happens again, if another established drug is found useful for fifty or more disorders by thousands of physicians, then the FDA *should* take this as a precedent.

Every once in a while, routine or no routine, a little common sense should be permitted. This is an extraordinary matter, vital to our health. If the FDA was set up to help the American public, here's a chance to do something great for them—with no one's feelings hurt except routine's.

12.

OBSERVATIONS ON PHT— EXPLORATION OF POSSIBLE NEW USES

It used to be that the word drug had a solid respectable meaning. But in recent years drug and abuse have been put together in the same sentence so often, without discrimination, that the word drug has come into disrepute. It's confusing, and a shame. Today people brag, just before they ascend, "I never took a drug in my life." As if St. Peter cared.

Good drugs are a cheerful feature of our society. We should stop tarring them with the same brush we use on the bad ones—and be grateful for them. With this general comment off my chest I would like to make some observations about PHT.

* * *

PHT would appear to be the most broadly useful drug in our pharmacopoeia (unless another is hidden in the literature). Paradoxically, this valuable feature, this versatility, has interfered with our understanding of the drug. The idea that one substance can have as many uses as PHT has been difficult to accept. And this is understandable. Not too long ago the thinking was a single drug for a single disorder.

A discussion of the basic mechanisms of action of PHT will help us understand how one drug can have so many uses.

A basic mechanism of action study was the first study to demonstrate that PHT might be a therapeutic substance. In 1938 Putnam and Merritt tested PHT on cats in which convulsions were induced by electricity. Of a large group of substances, including the best-known anticonvulsants, it was the most effective in controlling the convulsions. Putnam and Merritt said, Eureka! Maybe we have a superior antiepileptic drug.

They did. And not only was PHT the most effective anticonvulsant but it was found to have another remarkable property. Unlike previously used substances it achieved its therapy without sedation.

Let's go back to Putnam and Merritt's original study— and apply hindsight. Suppose, instead of inferring that PHT would help the epileptic, Putnam and Merritt had drawn a broader inference from their data. Suppose they had inferred that PHT worked against inappropriate electrical activity. That also would have been a correct inference—but with far broader implications. And the properties of PHT would not have been obscured by the label "anticonvulsant." Today basic mechanism scientists use broad terminology for PHT. They refer to it as a membrane stabilizer.

From the early basic mechanisms study of Toman, in 1949, PHT has been found to correct inappropriate electrical activity in groups of cells, and in individual cells. This includes nerve cells, brain cells, muscle cells, in fact, all types of cells that exhibit marked electrical activity. Whether a cell is made hyperexcitable by electrical impulse, calcium withdrawal, oxygen withdrawal, or by poisons, PHT has been shown to counteract this excitability. Further, it has been demonstrated that, in amounts that correct abnormal cell function, PHT does not affect normal function.*

When we understand that PHT is a substance that stabilizes the hyperactive cell, without affecting normal cell function, we see its therapeutic potential in the human body, a machine that runs on electrical impulse. It is estimated that there are a trillion cells in the body, tens of billions in the brain alone. Thinking is an electrical process, the rhythms of the heart are electrically regulated, the rhythms of the gut are electrically regulated, muscle movement is electrically regulated, messages of pain are electrically referred, and more.

It's important to know that after a cell has been stimulated to fire a few times it becomes potentiated, easier to fire than a normal cell. This is called post-tetanic potentiation. If the stimulation is continued, the cell starts to fire on its own, and continues to fire until its energy is depleted—post-tetanic afterdischarge. PHT has a modifying effect on post-tetanic potentiation and a correcting effect on post-tetanic afterdischarge. This may account for PHT's therapeutic effect on persistent and repetitive thinking and on unnecessary repetitive messages of pain.

* * *

* See *The Broad Range of Clinical Use of PHT,* '88—Stabilization of Bioelectrical Activity, p.89–97.

PHT has a number of properties which set it apart from most substances. For ten distinctive characteristics see *The Broad Range of Clinical Use of PHT*, '88. For purposes here we should consider several of these properties.

PHT is a non-habit-forming substance.* The desirability of a non-habit-forming drug that can calm and also relieve pain is apparent—it may be particularly useful during withdrawal from habit-forming substances.

PHT, in therapeutic amounts, has a calming effect without being a sedative. This characteristic is unusual, and clinical observations, supported by basic mechanisms studies, show that PHT does not affect normal function. Not only does PHT not sedate but it has been shown to improve concentration and effect a return of energy. This can be attributed, at least in part, to the fact that an overactive brain (hyperexcitable cells) wastes energy compounds.† One can conjecture that when thoughts with negative emotions are diminished, the effect of these "down" emotions is eliminated, and "psychic" energy may return.

Now that preventive medicine is being given more and more consideration, PHT may be of special interest because of its general properties and its versatility.

* * *

PHT, as do other drugs, has side effects. Safety and Toxicology of PHT is reviewed in *The Broad Range of Clinical Use of PHT*, '88. A replication of Parke-Davis's

---

* This is not to be confused with the well-known fact that a person with epilepsy should *not* abruptly discontinue PHT.

† PHT has been shown to increase energy compounds in the brain. See *The Broad Range of Clinical Use of PHT*, '88, p. 137.

package insert is included in the *Physicians' Desk Reference.* It should be noted that PHT is not on the Government's list of Controlled Drugs.

PHT can be used on a regular basis or on an occasional basis by the nonepileptic—depending on need. In the nonepileptic, effective doses tend to be lower than those used for epilepsy. The reader is reminded that PHT is a prescription drug and should be obtained from a physician.

* * *

When the Dreyfus Medical Foundation was preparing *The Broad Range of Use of Phenytoin,* in 1970, there were many published studies to draw on—1,900 by the time of publication. Seven hundred fifty references were selected and over 300 of them were summarized. These summaries were presented chronologically in order to show in sequence how the information about PHT developed.

Five years later when *PHT, 1975* was published, there were more than twice the number of studies to review, and the interrelationship between the clinical effects and basic mechanisms of action of PHT was in better perspective. In this bibliography the medical material was arranged according to subject matter for the convenience of the reader. Examples of this are found under such headings as Stabilization of Bioelectrical Activity, Anti-anoxic Effects, Anti-toxic Effects, Treatment of Pain, and others.

As an instance, under Anti-anoxic Effects of PHT, ten studies are grouped.* They were published in nine different journals, over a span of twenty years. Each of them is interesting but, by itself, would not carry much weight. But when these studies are reviewed together, the evi-

---

* This was in 1975. In the present Bibliography, 1988, there are forty-one studies.

dence that PHT has an offsetting effect against oxygen lack in animals is highly significant.

These basic studies furnish rationale for the clinical findings first made by Shulman in 1942, *New England Journal of Medicine*, that PHT is effective in asthma—and other studies in asthma, by Sayer and Polvan, *Lancet* (1968), and Shah, Vora, Karkhanis and Talwalkar, *Indian Journal of Chest Diseases* (1970).* They also furnish rationale for exploration of new uses.

* * *

Exploration of Possible New Uses

Since Putnam and Merritt's discovery in 1938 that phenytoin was a therapeutic substance, a steadily increasing number of uses for it have been found. The probabilities are high that there are more to come. Evidence from existing clinical and basic mechanisms of action studies furnishes clues for further exploration.

PHT has been reported effective in a wide variety of severely painful conditions.† Its usefulness as a non-habit-forming analgesic in milder forms of pain, and also in rheumatic conditions, and arthritis needs investigation.

The anti-anoxic effects of PHT point to its possible usefulness in stroke, emphysema, shock, and, in fact, in any condition where oxygen lack is a problem.

There are a number of references in the literature to beneficial effects of PHT on hypertension. Recently, in a

---

* The latter authors give an additional rationale, PHT's potential usefulness against the paroxysmal outbursts of asthma by its ability to stop post-tetanic afterdischarge.

† See *The Broad Range of Clinical Use of PHT*, '88, p. 48–55.

study of mildly hypertensive patients, treatment with PHT was reported effective.* Further study of PHT in hypertension, both by itself and in combination with hypertensive drugs, seems indicated.

A use of PHT that has received little attention, and that may have great potential, is its use topically, for the treatment of pain and for the promotion of healing.

Systemic PHT has been reported useful in healing in a variety of disorders—in leg ulcers, stomach ulcers, scleroderma, pruritus ani, and epidermolysis bullosa.†

The first report of a topical use of PHT was in 1972. Savini, Poitevin and Poitevin, *Revue Française d'Odonto-Stomatologie,* found topical PHT effective against pain and in the promotion of healing in periodontal disease. These findings were confirmed by three other studies in 1972 and by a double-blind study in 1977.

No study has been done by me but I have an obligation to report that I've seen PHT used topically, many times, on cuts, burns, bruises, and other surface conditions. From these informal observations it is apparent that PHT, used topically, is rapidly effective in the elimination of pain, and it would appear to shorten the time of healing. (Since this was written a recent controlled study of forty severely burned patients found that patients treated with topical PHT were able to receive skin grafts in less than half the time of patients conventionally treated.)‡

---

* See de la Torre, Murgia-Suarez and Aldrete, *The Broad Range of Clinical Use of PHT,* '88, p. 33.

† See *The Broad Range of Clinical Use of PHT,* '88, pp. 56–62.

‡ Mendiola-Gonzalez, Espejo-Plascencia, Chapa-Alvarez and Rodriguez-Noriega, *Investigacion Médica Internacional,* 10: 443–7, 1983.

Since the foregoing was written in 1981, there has been substantial evidence from at least four countries that, used topically, PHT is rapidly effective against the pain of burns, ulcers, wounds and other surface conditions, and that it speeds healing time. In the last year, its effectiveness against intractable ulcers of leprosy has been reported.

Other areas of investigation will suggest themselves to physicians.

13.
CONCLUSION
AND PERSONAL NOTE

"Truth is a precious thing and should be used sparingly."—Mark Twain. I have squandered a good deal of this precious commodity in writing this book—my supply is low—and it is time to conclude.

With the completion of this book I will have done what I can to communicate the facts about PHT. The Dreyfus Medical Foundation is going out of the communications business. It is not that we have lost interest, but to continue to argue the case for PHT could be counterproductive. This is a matter for others now.

Duplicates of the Foundation's extensive files on PHT are herewith offered to the Federal government. Access to these files will continue to be available to physicians. The Foundation intends to stay in the field of PHT and hopes, selectively, to sponsor research in new areas.

Thank you if you have read some of this book. And the best of everything to you. As for me, I am going to get in a rowboat and float upstream.

14.

THE ONE-HOUR TEST
Additional Chapter*

When the *Life* and *Reader's Digest* articles were published in 1967 there began a steady flow of people to the Dreyfus Medical Foundation. Many were struck by the similarity of the symptoms they had to symptoms I'd had, as described in the articles, and wanted to talk to me about it. After they'd gotten a prescription, I had the opportunity to talk with many of these people before they took their first PHT. These talks were beneficial to both of us, informative for them and educational for me.

I haven't kept exact count, no study as such was being done, but over the years I've talked with over two thousand persons before and after they've taken PHT. As a result of these talks, a test evolved. The test is in two parts. The first part deals with somatic conditions and is outlined at the end of this chapter. The second part deals with the effects of PHT on thoughts and emotions—in an explicit way. Because it differs from other tests, I will discuss it in some detail.

* * *

While I was in the depression, described earlier in this book, my brain was busy with thoughts I wanted to turn

* While writing the hardcover version of this book I considered including a one-hour test for PHT, but didn't. A number of physicians have told me that it should have been included. The test and how it came about is described here.

off but couldn't. These thoughts were invariably unhappy ones, mostly associated with fear, sometimes with anger. My brain worked on its own. It paid little attention to the landlord, I hesitate to use the word owner. When I took PHT this symptom disappeared, and I had an insight (in the literal sense) into the effects of PHT on thoughts and emotions. In those days I thought of this symptom as the "turned-on mind." It still seems an appropriate description and I will use it or the initials T.O.M.*

The turned-on mind is a symptom that most of us will identify with. Let me describe what I mean by it. We're told that we're always thinking about something. But "always thinking" can be misleading. There's a great difference between normal cerebration and abnormal. For example: You sit in the park relaxed, listening to the birds, enjoying the trees and smelling the grass. Beautiful, and healthy. Or, you sit in the park and your mind is so busy you're not even aware of the birds or the trees or the grass. This might be because you have a real problem. But if you don't have a real problem, then it's the turned-on mind.

My first opportunity to observe the T.O.M. closely was in the Worcester Jail study. Its effects were clear. The brains of the prisoners were so overactive that concentration was impaired. This interfered with reading. The subjects would see the words, but thoughts would intrude and they couldn't absorb what they read. They couldn't even remember what they'd seen on TV. The prisoners made it clear that their turned-on minds were busy with thoughts connected with the emotions of anger and fear. Obviously, with these emotions predominant, their mood was poor.

Subsequent experience showed that the T.O.M. is a

* I dislike making initials out of phrases but it's been the vogue since WW II.

common complaint with most of the people who need PHT. For years my only way of ascertaining this was by the straightforward question, "Do you have any thoughts now, other than what we are talking about, that you can't turn off?" Answers were usually in the affirmative. I got replies such as "I can't stop thinking for a minute," "My mind is like a five-ring circus," "My brain is going around and around." And similar comments. An hour after 100 mg of PHT, the same question got a different response. It was apparent that the over-thinking had quieted and mood had improved. But the change couldn't be measured. I would have liked to have had a more objective test.

One day I was talking to a young woman before she took her first 100 mg of PHT, and asked the standard question, "Is your brain busy with thoughts you can't turn off?" She said, "Oh yes, a lot of them." Something in the way she answered made me ask, "How many?" She said about fourteen. "Fourteen?" I said, and challengingly asked if she could write them down. I gave her pencil and pad and almost without pause she wrote down twelve thoughts. I was astonished that she could locate these thoughts and write them down. It didn't occur to me to ask her questions about the thoughts.

An hour after PHT, I again asked if she could write down her thoughts. She said she could—this time there were just two. One of them was, "I am angry with my mother." Earlier, she had written, "I am very, very angry with my mother." With PHT her mother was two very's better off.

The following day I met with a man I'd known for several years. Jim was thirty-five and had a lot going for him. But he said he was depressed. PHT had been prescribed and he wanted to talk with me before taking it.

These were Jim's circumstances as he related them. He was doing so well in his work that he was leaving a firm he'd been with for years to go into business for himself. The firm had been good to him and he felt badly about leaving. Also, there was a change in his private life. He had fallen in love with another woman and was leaving his wife and two children to get married again. It was a mixed bag. There were things to be happy about, and there were realistic concerns.

As with the young woman the day before, I asked Jim if he could write down the thoughts he couldn't turn off. He considered for a moment and then wrote steadily. When he finished, he said there were nine thoughts. (See column on the left, below.)

At that point I asked a question I'd never asked before. I asked Jim to think of the first thought on his list, and if any emotions came with it to write them down. He thought, and then wrote. I asked him to repeat the procedure with the second thought, and so on.

This is the list of Jim's thoughts and the emotions attached to them. When he handed it to me he volunteered, " 'Unfocus' is the worst problem in my life."

With his thoughts and emotions in writing, Jim took 100 mg of PHT. Not wanting my presence to have a possible effect, I left him to his own devices for an hour. When I rejoined him I gave him a fresh piece of paper and asked the same questions. This time he wrote:

Job   — Success · Guilt
Girl   — Love —
Money   — ?
Wife   — Sadness

When he finished Jim looked at what he'd written and had a belly laugh. He said, isn't that a typical American boy's story—JOB, GIRL, MONEY, WIFE. I report the laugh because there weren't any laughs in Jim an hour earlier.

This was the first complete one-hour test for thoughts and emotions. It is a good test for illustration purposes; it demonstrates three points:

One. A striking diminution of extraneous and unnecessary thoughts is seen within an hour after PHT. These thoughts are usually accompanied by emotions related to anger and fear.* When the thoughts disappear, the negative emotions disappear with them.

Two. The PHT needer has poor concentration and is unlikely to remember what his condition was before he took PHT. That is why it is necessary to get things down in writing. Before taking PHT, Jim said that "unfocus" was his worst problem. An hour later I asked, "What is your worst problem?" Jim couldn't remember "unfocus."

Three. PHT does not cause realistic concerns to go away. Jim had two real problems. They were still there but in better perspective. After PHT he still felt guilt in leaving his firm, but now "guilt" was coupled with "success" (he was starting his own business). He still had realistic concern about his family, but instead of *children (guilt, remorse)* this was moderated to *wife (sadness)*.†

Let me re-emphasize that the test should be done in writing. People who need PHT are poor observers and are almost sure to forget how they were an hour before.

* * *

* Note that on Jim's first list, with the exception of love, all the emotions are related to anger and fear.

† This was the first of many hundreds of such tests. These tests were not "controlled" by placebo or other drugs. The persons were taking PHT for therapeutic reasons and that was out of the question. However, there was an interesting element of control.

Initially, I wasn't sure how long it took for PHT to become effective and I experimented with repeating the questions at different time intervals, including five and ten minutes after PHT. In these two time periods I never saw positive results. On the other hand, beneficial effects of PHT were always seen between forty-five minutes and one hour.

This was a useful control. A suggestible person (placebo responder) would be as apt to respond in ten minutes. On the other hand, for all to respond within the same narrow time frame, and it not be due to PHT, would strain the laws of coincidence.

Everybody's talking at me
I don't hear a word they're saying
Only the echoes of my mind.
            —"Everybody's Talking,"
                        Midnight Cowboy

"Only the echoes of my mind." What a beautiful and perceptive line. To a lesser or greater degree it describes the PHT needer.

Until this test evolved it wouldn't have occurred to me that a person could identify the thoughts alive in his brain, think of them singly, and write down the emotions that came with them. I'd always thought of "echoes of my mind" as being unconscious or subconscious. I still think they are—most of the time. But when a specific question is asked, the echoes become conscious and can be identified. Thus the same questions, asked before and after PHT, enable one to compare quantitative changes in thoughts and qualitative changes in emotions.

When you have seen the response to this test over and over again, you start to think of the thoughts as kites and the emotions that come with them as the tails of the kites. When the thoughts disappear, the tail (the negative emotions) disappears with them. Deeper consideration of this point makes one realize that sometimes the negative emotion (the tail) may come first. When that happens the emotion (of chemical or bioelectrical origin) can always find a thought to attach itself to. But PHT does not care for these niceties. Whether the tail or the kite comes first, improvement an hour after PHT is marked.

A majority of PHT needers have persistent thoughts they can't turn off. A small minority do not have persistent thoughts, but a jumble of thoughts flashing in and out. Both conditions are corrected or improved within an hour. The effects of PHT are so consistent that it helps to remember that, in the laboratory, PHT always corrects post-tetanic afterdischarge. It makes no exceptions, regardless of the type of nerve or the cause of excitation.

The turned-on mind is not just a daytime phenomenon. It continues at night and can make it difficult to fall asleep. It can also be the cause of light sleep filled with unpleasant dreams and frequent nightmares. That is why PHT's effectiveness against the turned-on mind is helpful with sleeping problems.

Only two more tests will be discussed here. One test was with a woman who used to be seen frequently on television. You could call her an intellectual, in a nice way. Before she took PHT, I asked if she had any thoughts, other than what we were talking about, alive in her head. "Oh, I always do," she said. "Doesn't everyone?" Then she wrote down seven thoughts she couldn't turn off. All of them were connected with worries and concerns. When she finished she said, "I always have music playing in my head. It's like a jukebox and I can tell you what record is on."

An hour after taking PHT, before I could ask any questions, this woman volunteered that she was trying to be objective but she didn't think PHT had any effect. Again, I asked if there were any thoughts that she couldn't turn off. She said no—in the most matter-of-fact way. I said, "What is playing in your jukebox now?" She said, "Nothing." That woke her up, and she exclaimed, "My goodness, I feel like a weight is off my chest." *

* This sort of comment is not uncommon. When negative emotions are relieved, people tend to become more lighthearted and have a return of energy.

One other test. It was with a physician who was doing research on PHT. He mentioned that he had been sleeping badly and that he was a little depressed. I suggested it might be useful for him to try PHT, both for personal reasons and also for research purposes. He agreed.

After I asked him the standard question* he started writing down the thoughts "alive" in his brain. He wrote and wrote. When he had written twenty-six, he paused for a moment and looked up. I said that's enough, Fred, you've already set a record. Now go back to the first thought, think of it for a moment, and write the emotion or emotions that come with it.

For our purposes, and to save space, I'll leave out the thoughts and just show the last twelve emotions.

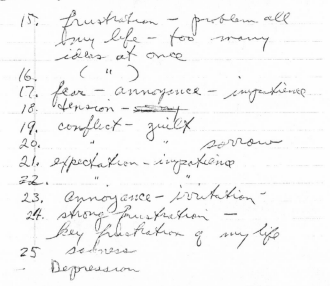

15. frustration — problem all
my life — too many
ideas at once
16. (")
17. fear — annoyance — impatience
18. tension —
19. conflict — guilt
20. " " sorrow
21. expectation — impatience
22. " "
23. annoyance — irritation —
24. strong frustration —
key frustration of my life
25. sadness
— Depression

---

* It can be helpful to start with the question, "Do you remember what you had for breakfast?" When the subject tells you, you explain, "You weren't thinking of that until I asked. You got it out of your memory. That is *not* the type of thought we're interested in. What we want to know is, are there any thoughts alive in your head going on now?"

Fred took 100 mg of PHT. An hour later I asked the same questions. He wrote:

1. *Lunch in sun - pleasant place to relax*

2. *Coffee was good this morning*

3. *No noticeable effect of PHT*

When I read No. 3, "No noticeable effect of PHT," I thought he was putting me on. But I saw he was serious. I said, "Fred, get out the list you wrote an hour ago." He looked at the list—and it all came back to him. He wrote:

No neck, shoulder, or back tension or pain -

Feeling tone pleasant - anticipating sitting in sun at lunch.

Depression seems entirely gone

Relaxed! - not overwhelmed by multiple, simultaneous thoughts or ideas.

at peace with myself -

The turned-on mind is usually occupied with the same thoughts, repeated over and over again. This last test illustrates a less frequent condition—a confusion of thoughts flashing in and out. As Fred described it, "frustration—problem all my life—too many ideas at once."

* * *

The one-hour test is in two parts. As to the somatic part of the test: No person has all of the listed symptoms, but three, four, or more are not uncommon. An hour after PHT, moderation or elimination of symptoms is usually observed.

As to the second part of the test: Unnecessary thoughts are usually diminished in one hour and the negative emotions that come with them are decreased or eliminated. This is a more objective method of assessing changes in mood than asking "How do you feel?" before PHT and again an hour later.

(Outline of the One-Hour Test is on the next two pages.)

THE ONE-HOUR TEST

Part I—Somatic Conditions

These questions pertain to how you feel now. If you answer yes to any question, grade your symptom, on a scale of 1–10 (1, minimal; 10, most severe).

	Before PHT	*After PHT*
Do you have a headache of any sort?	_____	_____
Any pain or blurring in the eyes?	_____	_____
Any ache or pain in the neck?	_____	_____
In the shoulders, the back, or chest?	_____	_____
Shortness of breath?	_____	_____
Aches or pains in your arms or hands?	_____	_____
Aches or pains in your legs or feet?	_____	_____
Are your hands or feet hot or cold?	_____	_____
Any tingling sensations?	_____	_____
Any "knots" or "butterflies" in your stomach?	_____	_____
Are you trembling now? Hold out your hands and observe.	_____	_____
Do you feel any trembling inside?	_____	_____
Do you feel a pulse, or beat, or throb inside you?	_____	_____
How is your energy now?	_____	_____
Do you have any pain or discomfort not asked about?	_____	_____

Part II—Thoughts and Emotions

It is useful to begin by asking the patient what he had for breakfast. When he tells you, remind him that he got the answer from his memory, it wasn't "alive" in his brain. Explain that's not what you want. What you are looking for are thoughts that are going on right now, that are difficult to turn off.

If there are such thoughts, ask the patient to write them on the left side of a piece of paper, explaining that you don't need to see them since they might be personal. It's the emotions that come with the thoughts that you want. Then ask the patient to think each thought separately, and write opposite it the emotions that come with it. Do this for each thought.

An hour after 100 mg of PHT, ask the same questions again.

Before PHT

THOUGHTS   EMOTIONS

_____   _____

_____   _____

_____   _____

_____   _____

_____   _____

_____   _____

_____   _____

_____   _____

_____   _____

After PHT

_____   _____

_____   _____

_____   _____

_____   _____

APPENDIX

Symptoms and Disorders For Which PHT Has Been Reported Useful

Anger (impatience, irritability)
Angina pectoris
Arthritis
Asthma
Cardiac arrhythmias
Cardiac conduction defect
Cerebrovascular insufficiencies
Choreoathetosis
Cognitive function (ruminative thinking, concentration, learning disability)
Continuous muscle fiber activity (myokymia, myotonia, etc.)
Depression
Diabetic neuropathy
Drug and alcohol withdrawal
Dysesthesias
Eating disorders (anorexia, bulimia)
Epidermolysis bullosa
Fear (anxiwty, tension)
Fever
Head injury
Healing (systemic and topical)

Hyperkinesia
Hypertension
Hypoglycemia
Irritable bowel syndrome
Intractable hiccups
Labile diabetes
Migraine and other headaches
Muscle spasms
Myocardial infarction
Overthinking
Pain
Parkinson's syndrome
Pruritus ani
Q-T interval syndrome
Scleroderma
Sleep disorders
Stuttering
Surgery (pre- and postoperative)
Tinnitus
Toxic effects of other drugs
Trigeminal neuralgia and other neuralgias
Violent behavior

Medical Journals In Which Many of the
Clinical Uses of PHT Have Been Reported

Acta Dermato-Venereologica
Acta Endocrinologica
Acta Medica Scandinavica
Acta Neurologica
Acta Neurologica Scandinavica
Acta Medica Venezolana
Actualités Odonto-
  Stomatologiques
American Heart Journal
American Journal of Cardiology
American Journal of Diseases of
  Children
American Journal of Digestive
  Diseases
American Journal of the
  Medical Sciences
American Journal of Medicine
American Journal of Physiology
American Journal of Psychiatry
American Journal of
  Psychotherapy
American Journal of Surgery
Anales de Medicina de
  Barcelona
Anaesthesia and Intensive Care
Anesthesia and Analgesia
Anesthesiology
Angiology
Annales de Cardiologie et
  d'Angeiologie
Annales de Dermatologie et de
  Syphiligraphie
Annales de Medecine Interne
Annals of Emergency Medicine
Annals of Internal Medicine
Annals of Neurology
Annals of Rheumatic Diseases
Antiseptic
Archiv für Ohren-, Nasen- und
  Kehlkopfheilkunde
Archives of Dermatology

Archives of General Psychiatry
Archives of Internal Medicine
Archives des Maladies du Coeur
  et des Vaisseaux
Archives of Neurology
Archives of Neurology and
  Psychiatry
Archives of Otolaryngology
Archives of Pediatrics
Archives of Physical Medicine
  and Rehabilitation
Archives of Surgery
Archivos del Instituto de
  Cardiologia de México
Arquivos de Neuro-Psiquiatria
Arteriosclerosis
Arthritis and Rheumatism
Arztliche Wochenschrift
Australian Journal of
  Dermatology
Biulleten Vsesoiuznogo
  Kardiologicheskogo
  Nauchnogo (Moscow)
Blut
Brain
British Heart Journal
British Journal of Addiction
British Journal of Clinical
  Pharmacology
British Journal of Dermatology
British Journal of Radiology
British Medical Journal
Bulletin of the Los Angeles
  Neurological Societies
Bulletin of the New York
  Academy of Medicine
California Medicine
Canadian Anaesthetists Society
  Journal
Canadian Medical Association
  Journal

Canadian Psychiatric
　　Association Journal
Ceskoslovenska Neurologie
Chest
Child's Brain
China Medical Abstracts
Chinese Medical Journal
Circulation
Clinical
　　Electroencephalography
Clinical Journal of Pain
Clinical Medicine
Clinical Nephrology
Clinical Neurology
Clinical Neuropharmacology
Clinical Neurophysiology
Clinical Pharmacology and
　　Therapeutics
Clinical Research
Clinical Science
Clinical Science and Molecular
　　Medicine
Clinical Therapeutics
Clinician
Comprehensive Psychiatry
Connecticut Medicine
Criminal Psychopathology
Critical Care Medicine
Current Therapeutic
　　Research
Cutis
Delaware Medical Journal
Dental Hygiene
Deutsche Medizinische
　　Wochenschrift
Deutsche Stomatologie
Diabetes
Diseases of the Chest
Diseases of the Nervous System
Ear, Nose and Throat Journal
Electroencephalography and
　　Clinical Neurophysiology
Epilepsia
European Journal of Clinical
　　Investigation

European Journal of Clinical
　　Pharmacology
European Neurology
Experimental Medicine and
　　Surgery
Fertility and Sterility
Folia Psychiatrica et
　　Neurologica Japonica
Fortschritte der Neurologie-
　　Psychiatrie
Gaceta Medica Española
Gastroenterologie Clinique et
　　Biologique
Gastroenterology
Geriatrics
Giornale de Psichiatria e di
　　Neuropatologia
Handchirurgie, Mikrochirurgie,
　　Plastische Chirurgie
Harefuah
Hautarzt
Headache
HNO-Praxis
Indian Journal of Chest
　　Diseases
Intensive Care Medicine
International Journal of
　　Dermatology
International Journal of
　　Neuropsychiatry
International Surgery
Investigacion Medica
　　Internacional
Israel Journal of Medical
　　Sciences
Italian Journal of Neurological
　　Sciences
Johns Hopkins Medical
　　Journal
Journal of American College of
　　Cardiology
Journal of the American
　　Geriatrics Society
Journal of the American
　　Medical Association

Journal of the American
  Osteopathic Association
Journal of the Association of
  Physicians in India
Journal of Cardiovascular
  Surgery
Journal of Clinical
  Endocrinology and
  Metabolism
Journal of Clinical
  Investigation
Journal of Clinical
  Pharmacology
Journal of Clinical
  Psychiatry
Journal of Dermatologic
  Surgery and Oncology
Journal of Diabetic Association
  of India
Journal of the Egyptian Medical
  Association
Journal of Emergency Medicine
Journal of the Florida Medical
  Association
Journal of Formosan Medical
  Association
Journal of the Indian Medical
  Association
Journal of the Kansas Medical
  Society
Journal of Laboratory and
  Clinical Medicine
Journal of Laryngology and
  Otology
Journal of Mental Science
Journal of the Michigan State
  Medical Society
Journal of the Mississippi State
  Medical Association
Journal of Nervous and Mental
  Disease
Journal of the National
  Proctologic Association
Journal of Neurology
Journal of Neurology,

Neurosurgery and
  Psychiatry
Journal of Neurosurgery
Journal of Neurosurgical
  Sciences
Journal of Oral Surgery
Journal of Orthomolecular
  Psychiatry
Journal of Pediatrics
Journal of Reproductive
  Medicine
Journal of Rheumatology
Journal of Surgery
Journal of Urology
Kardiologiia
Klinische Wochenschrift
Lancet
Laryngoscope
Lyon Medical
Maryland Medical Journal
Medical Clinics of North
  America
Medical Journal of Australia
Medicina Cutanea Ibero-Latino-
  Americana
Medicina Experimentalis
Medizinische Klinik
Medizinische Monatsschrift
Metabolism
Michigan Medicine
Minerva Cardioangiologica
Modern Concepts of
  Cardiovascular Disease
Monatsschrift Psychiatric and
  Neurologie
Mount Sinai Medical Journal
Münchener Medizinische
  Wochenschrift
Muscle and Nerve
Nebraska State Medical Journal
Nederlands Tijdschrift Voor
  Geneeskunde
Nervenarzt
Neurologia i Neurochirurgia
  Polska

Neurologia Medico-Chirurgica
Neurology
Neuropadiatrie
Neuropsychobiology
Neurosurgery
Neurosurgical Science
New England Journal of
    Medicine
New York State Journal of
    Medicine
New Zealand Medical Journal
Pacing and Clinical
    Electrophysiology
Pediatrics
Physician's Drug Manual
Pittsburgh Medical Bulletin
Polish Medical Journal
Polski Tygodnik Lekarsky
Portsmouth Journal of
    Psychology
Postgraduate Medical Journal
Postgraduate Medicine
Practitioner
Prensa Medica Argentina
Presse Medicale
Problemy Endokrinologii
Proceedings of American
    Association of Cancer
    Research
Proceedings of the Australian
    Association of Neurologists
Proceedings of the Symposium
    on Aggressive Behavior
Progress in Cardiovascular
    Disease
Psychiatric Journal of the
    University of Ottawa
Psychopharmacologia
Psychophysiology
Psychosomatic Medicine
Psychosomatics
Rational Drug Therapy
Revista Argentina de
    Cardiologia
Revista Brasileira de
    Anestesiologia

Revista Clinica Española
Revista Española de
    Pediatria
Revista Iberica de
    Endocrinologia
Revista de Medicina
    Interna
Revue de Laryngologie
Revue Medicale de Liege
Revue de Médecine
    Aeronautique et Spatiale
Revue Neurologique
Revue d'Odonto-Stomatologie
Revue d'Oto-Neuro-
    Ophthalmologie
Revue Roumaine de Medecine
    Serie Neurologie et
    Psychiatrie
Rivista di Neurologia
Russian Pharmacology and
    Toxicology
Schweizerische Medizinische
    Wochenschrift
Semaine des Hospitaux
South African Journal of
    Laboratory and Clinical
    Medicine
South African Medical Journal
Southern Medical Journal
Stomatologie der DDR
Stroke
Svensk Larkartidningen
Therapeutic Archives
Therapeutic Drug Monitoring
Therapeutische Umschau
Therapiewoche
Transactions of the American
    Neurological Association
Vrachebnoe Delo
Virginia Medical Monthly
Vnitrni Lekarstvi
Western Medicine
Wiener Klinische Wochenschrift
Zeitschrift fur Hautkrankheiten
Zhurnal Nevropatologii i
    Psikhiatrii Korsakova

Early Cases

The cases of the third, fourth, fifth, and sixth persons I saw take Dilantin (PHT) are summarized. The names have been changed.

THIRD CASE. Elizabeth Brown. Came from Miami to New York for diagnosis. She couldn't turn off her thoughts and was depressed, agitated, and filled with fear. Was diagnosed in New York by a colleague of Dr. Silbermann's as a schizoid type. PHT was tried. It had been thought she would need a companion to take her back to Miami, but her improvement on PHT was such that the physicians felt it was not necessary. In Miami she was treated by Dr. A. Lester Stepner. A letter from Dr. Stepner stated: "She had suffered from a depression and had suicidal thoughts. She had not been able to function in any constructive manner. She is now taking Dilantin regularly and feels that this has controlled the impulsive acts which have made it difficult for her to keep her job. She is not depressed, has passed the intensive courses of the airline stewardess, and is now working for National Airlines."

FOURTH CASE. George Lewis. George, a business associate of mine, came to see me about an office procedure. I didn't agree with the procedure he liked, but when I saw how important it was to him I agreed to do it his way. He continued to argue his point, and I realized he hadn't even heard me. I asked him how he felt. He said he was depressed and worried all the time, and for the last few weeks had only slept a couple of hours a night. I sent him to Dr. Silbermann who put him on PHT, on a Friday. When I saw him on Monday he was in a good mood and had slept soundly Saturday and Sunday. He stopped taking PHT on his own, and in a few days his mood deteriorated. He took PHT again and an hour later volunteered, "I've got my strength back! I've got my strength." He continued the medicine with good effect.

In the next two cases, which I couldn't follow closely, I asked the subjects to write me their experiences.

FIFTH CASE. Mary Jones. Excerpts from her letter:

I was in a state of uneasiness and an undefinable morbid fear accompanied me. A good night's sleep seemed the most elusive of luxuries.

After taking Dilantin for two or three days, I started to feel much better. A calm came over me and I was free from that inner disturbance. What a relief from that nervous jerky feeling I had when I endeavored to do the simplest things. What is really marvelous is that I sleep at night. No longer do I stay awake manufacturing problems.

Then I stopped taking PHT. What a change came over me! Saturday I was depressed and by Saturday evening I was in rare form. Listening to *Tosca*, I started on a crying jag that lasted throughout the night.

After three days of that nonsense, I started taking Dilantin again on Tuesday. I started feeling much better. By the way, I'm now making a test—*Tosca* is on and I feel great!

SIXTH CASE. Evelyn Smith. Excerpts from her letter:

I want to express my feelings as much as possible before I started taking PHT.

I had become a really sick person. I had got so disgusted with life that I hated people. I started staying by myself, not going anywhere, not doing anything. I couldn't even stand going shopping. I wanted to sleep to escape, but I couldn't sleep. Then I started taking sleeping pills, and I stopped eating and lost weight. I would have periods of deep depression.

Then I started taking PHT. I remember no reactions as far as a sleeping pill or anything similar makes you feel, but I started taking an interest in life again. After two or three days I noticed that I could drive my car and traffic didn't upset me anymore. Matter of fact I was relaxed, enjoying listening to the car radio.

Then I noticed that waiters and people around me didn't bother me anymore.

I have no trouble sleeping now, and I've stopped taking sleeping pills. Now I can talk to someone or read a book without a million thoughts creeping up and crushing what I am thinking about.

I have gained eight pounds and weigh 106. I am happier than I have ever been that I can remember. And my friends have noticed the change in me, for many have mentioned it.

Transcripts of Seven Cases
Worcester County Jail Study

JOHN G.

Before PHT:

I'm nervous, irritable, and I brood a lot over things that are already over and done with. I make more of them inside which keeps me in quite a state of nervousness, anger, tension, what have you.

I magnify everything to the extent where I make myself uncomfortable . . . I'm never relaxed enough to take time to try to figure out what makes me move—I can't control myself and I just don't seem to give a damn one way or the other.

With PHT (Non-Blind):

I'm quite relaxed. I feel good.

I slept real good . . . I'm not as worked up so I stay awake . . . When it's bedtime, I'm ready to go.

I'm more easygoing . . . I'm not as short with the fellas as I usually am . . . I've only blown my top once . . . It just lasted a few seconds . . . I didn't brood about it afterwards.

After Being Off PHT (Two Weeks):

Before I took the medicine, I felt the same way as I do now . . . More or less quick to jump. In fact, a lot of times I might jump before I think it over.

I've had two good arguments since I've been off the medication.

I've had a few headaches in the morning . . . A lot of times I have a headache during the day when I get worked up over something.

I'm not sleeping. I wouldn't say I'm sleeping sound at all . . . I'm having some dreams . . . they are very unpleasant . . . and uncomfortable, tiring.

With PHT (Double-Blind):

I think I'm improved all over . . . An hour after I took the pill I could have told you it wasn't sugar . . . You could feel the engine just slowing right down.

I'm very relaxed and I'm not uncomfortable in any way . . . I can sort of think ahead.

I been sleeping soundly, no trouble, no lying awake thinking about things. That's more or less what kept me awake; the brain was overactive . . . but now I just drop right off.

I still have anger but I don't blow up . . . Quite a bit of restraint which I never had . . . The anger doesn't hang on like it did before.

VICTOR M.

Before PHT:

Well, I am nervous. I bite my fingernails. I got a nervous disorder . . . my hands shake . . . I have a lot of headaches and a pain in the stomach all the time.

I don't go to sleep till about one or two o'clock in the morning . . . I toss around a lot . . . I could put the blanket over me and sometimes find the blanket on the floor.

My mind must be busy . . . I can't turn it off.

With PHT (Non-Blind):

I'm sleeping better . . . I sleep right through and don't get up any more like I used to.

I feel better than I did . . . I don't feel that nervous now . . .

About the pain in my stomach, I don't get it as often as I used to
. . . I don't get headaches as much.

I'm not as grouchy as I used to be . . . Now very often I don't
get mad.

After Being Off PHT (Two Weeks):
When I was taking the pills I felt better and now, after I
came off the pills, I don't feel so good . . . I'm restless.

I can't sleep.

I get in my cell and I won't even come out.

With PHT (Double-Blind):
I'm in a good mood . . . I wasn't angry all week long . . .
I didn't have any arguments with anyone.

Right now I've been sleeping more than before . . . Every
afternoon, pretty near, I take a nap.

The pain in my stomach went away . . . I haven't had a headache all week . . . I haven't been biting my nails.

ALTON B.

Before PHT:
I'm pretty nervous . . . I feel a little shaky all over.

My stomach is all tied up . . . It feels like it's all twisted up.
Bothered me quite a lot lately.

I've been having headaches.

At the end of the day I get worn out.

With PHT (Non-Blind):
I feel pretty good for a change . . . I don't feel shaky . . . I
feel more relaxed.

I don't think too much . . . it seems like I have more patience
. . . I sit down and watch television for one program. I never
could do that before.

I guess I been sleepin' better . . . When I wake up in the
morning my head feels clearer than it did before.

My stomach don't feel like it's all tied up . . . I can eat good.

I haven't had any headaches and I'm not so tired.

After Being Off PHT (Two Weeks):
    I have been feeling nervous . . . I feel like I'm going right back where . . . like a nervous stomach and like I was before.
    Right now I'm rundown and I'm tired . . . no pep, no nothing.

With Placebo (Double-Blind):
    I feel miserable, lousy, tired, rundown . . . I feel shaky.

With PHT (Single-Blind):
    I don't know what the pill was, but I'm pretty sure it helped me.
    I feel pretty good . . . I feel cheerful . . . I feel good all over, I guess.

ALBERT M.

Before PHT:
    I get depressed very easily . . . Nothing seems good to me . . . I don't care what happens . . . I don't care if they put me in the hole, put me in solitary confinement.
    I'm quick-tempered . . . I hold back sometimes . . . the thought keeps harping, keeps harping . . . it stays longer than I like.
    If I get excited . . . if I get mad . . . I'll start shakin' . . . my whole body is goin'.

With PHT (Non-Blind):
    I feel more relaxed . . . I don't feel as much tension as I had.
    I haven't got angry . . . don't wake up grouchy like I used to.
    As far as headaches, I haven't had a headache now for about three days.

After Being Off PHT (Two Weeks):
    When I come off the pills I get depressed, very depressed. Headaches, anger, not eating well, not sleeping well . . . Nervous, very nervous.

With Placebo (Double-Blind):
   I didn't get to sleep till about three o'clock this morning and I was up about five-thirty.
   I'm worried . . . I don't know what's going to happen, but I don't think I can do any more time. It's really got me down. It's really got me depressed.
   Everything galls me. I just don't care for anything.

With PHT (Single-Blind):
   I'm pretty steady, sleepin' good, my appetite has come back . . . I'm not angry, not a bit. I was down-and-out. Since I been back on the medicine I feel pretty good.

WILFRED S.

Before PHT:
   Once in a while I just feel scared . . . I have a bad habit of biting my fingernails and biting my lip.
   I'm quick-tempered. I always want to keep on the move. I pace the floor, it seems to make me feel better if I just keep moving.
   I seem to think all the time. I have a hard time sleeping. I toss and turn for about an hour and wake up sometimes in the middle of the night from nightmares.

With PHT (Non-Blind):
   I feel fine . . . I haven't been nervous. I don't find myself thinking like I used to . . . I don't think as heavy.
   I haven't been scared, and I don't get in so many fights and arguments . . . I get along with the other fellas.
   I've been sleeping good . . . haven't had nightmares like I did before . . . feel more awake . . . I'm just not so tired.

After Being Off PHT (Two Weeks):
   Well, since I've been off the pills, I've seemed to tire more easily, I don't sleep too well at night and I'm more nervous now. And I notice myself quick-tempered.
   I do a lot more thinking now.

I've noticed the last couple of days I've slacked down on my eating. I don't have too much of an appetite.

With Placebo (Double-Blind):
I'm nervous all the time, very quick-tempered, feel depressed, feel tired.

I think constantly. I try to stop but I can't . . . I sort of keep thinking of different things all at the same time . . . I tend to think of other things at the same time I'm reading . . . I have a hard time remembering what I read.

With PHT (Single-Blind):
Well, it seems like all of a sudden I'm coming back to life . . .
My mood is much better. I don't get in so many arguments . . . I'm not so hot-tempered.

I can understand things better and concentrate on things. I don't have that continuous thinking. I'm not so tired because my mind isn't running all over the place.

ROBERT B.

Before PHT:
I would say I'm nervous . . . I have my fears. I get mad fast . . .

My mind is turned on . . . I go in my cell, I sit down and I start thinking. Many things go through my mind . . . and I work myself up and this can go on for a whole day . . . The only way I could probably turn it off is if somebody started talking to me . . . As soon as I stopped talking . . . it would just start up again.

I have a lot of trouble with sleeping . . . I wake up frequently.

I think I get very easily depressed . . . Many times a day. When anything doesn't go my way I get very depressed . . . I sulk. I don't talk to anybody and nobody can talk to me.

With PHT (Non-Blind):
I'm in a very good frame of mind . . . I just feel relaxed and

comfortable . . . The feeling that I got now is that I can sit here and listen to you talk rather than me talk to you.

I'm much calmer . . . And I noticed that the days go quicker. I didn't have any run-ins with anybody. Nothing bothered me.

I seem to have a clear outlook and everything seems to be sharper for me. I seem to be able to concentrate better . . . My mind just doesn't seem to be wandering as much.

After Being Off PHT (Two Weeks):

I feel lousy . . . very edgy, constant depression most of the time . . . I'm just not interested in anything . . . I have no desire to do anything.

I tried sleeping all morning, laying down, reading a book, but I just couldn't sleep. And I'm not getting that good a night's sleep.

I go from one subject to another . . . I have a lot of trouble writing a letter. I guess my mind wanders so much that as I'm writing a sentence out I completely forget what I'm writing about.

With PHT (Double-Blind):

I have no nervousness, no depression, no trouble with sleep. I just feel great.

I'm in a good frame of mind . . . I've been pretty calm, cool and collected. Happy.

I feel pretty lively . . . I have the feeling I want to do something . . . I don't have that tired, dragged-out feeling.

DANNY R.
ASSESSMENT OF DOUBLE-BLIND

In ten of the eleven cases, the investigators, and the subjects themselves, correctly assessed who was on PHT. The assessment of the eleventh case was complicated by a realistic problem that developed during the study which the subject did not tell us about, and the effects of PHT were masked by a realistic reaction. This was the case of Danny R. Before the problem arose, Danny R.'s response to PHT was similar to that of the other subjects. Danny R.'s realistic response to his problem, even with PHT, lends support to the description of PHT as a normalizer.

At the beginning of the study, on PHT, Danny R. reported that he slept sounder, that nervousness and excessive anger disappeared, energy returned, muscular pains in his shoulders went away and his mood improved. He illustrated improvement in concentration:

> DANNY R: I started a book yesterday. It's five hundred and some pages. I read about three hundred and fifty of them. I got locked in the bakery. Everybody left and I was still reading. I'm usually the first one out, see? I can concentrate now.

Then a serious question of his daughter's eyesight arose and Danny R. wrote home five times asking about his daughter and received no reply. He explains:

> DANNY R: Well, you mail a letter and you don't hear nothin'. Then you mail another one. You can't find out nothin'. You get in your cell at night, you start wonderin' is the baby going to lose an eye . . . You toss around half the night.
>
> JACK D: When we saw you Monday morning, you were nervous.
>
> DANNY R: Right.
>
> JACK D: We noticed it and we assumed that you were on placebo. Then we put you on a pill. You didn't know what it was, but we knew it was Dilantin. After we saw you, you received a letter from home. Well, you explain about the letter.
>
> DANNY R: The head runner give me a letter from my sister. She told me that my wife had said that the baby was all right and they were both doing fine. I felt good about it.

JACK D: Dan, you've had two experiences with the pill. The first one was for about a week. Do you think it helped you then?

DANNY R: It helped me. I know it did. You see, when I went into that first week, my nerves about normal for me . . . That week I was sleeping good, as I told you before. My hands were steadier. And I stayed out of trouble.

JACK D: Your anger was down?

DANNY R: Right.

JACK D: But this week, seemingly, the realistic problems overburdened the medicine. We don't know how you would have reacted without the pills.

DANNY R: If I wasn't taking them, truthfully, I think I would be in the state hospital right now. That's how bad I was.

JACK D: Okay, Dan. Thanks. Perhaps for the sake of this study it is just as well we had one miss, because nobody would believe it if we got everything right.

Lyman and Patuxent Studies

LYMAN

The study at the Lyman Reformatory for Boys was done with six boys aged eleven to thirteen, and the results were similar to those seen at the Worcester Jail. Five of the boys were moody and belligerent. After PHT they became friendly and smiling, and their fights decreased from five or sixth a day to one or two. The sixth boy was obviously depressed when we first saw him. We had a hard time even getting a *yes* or *no* from him. He never got into fights and stayed apart from the other boys. After he had taken PHT, he became loquacious and started having the "normal" one or two fights a day. The disparate effects of PHT, the calming effect on the boys that needed calming, and the return of energy to the depressed boys were interesting to observe.

PATUXENT

The Patuxent Institution was different from the Worcester County Jail. Unlike the inmates at Worcester, the prisoners at Patuxent had been convicted of the most serious crimes. But PHT made no distinction and the effects on the nervous systems of the five prisoners studied were similar to those observed at Worcester.

As a result of observations made during this study, Dr. Joseph Stephens conducted two double-blind studies with outpatients at Johns Hopkins and found PHT effective in reducing symptoms relating to fear and anger.*

---

* See Stephens and Shaffer, *Psychopharmacologia*, 1970, and Stephens and Shaffer, *J. Clin. Pharmacol.*, 1973, *The Broad Range of Clinical Use of PHT*, p. 7 and 9.

Secretary of HEW Elliot L. Richardson's Response to Inquiry from Governor Nelson A. Rockefeller

June 22, 1972

Dear Governor Rockefeller:

Please forgive the delay of this response to your April 19 letter concerning the current status of the drug, phenytoin.

Conversations with health officials within the Department have revealed that phenytoin (PHT) was introduced in 1938 as the first essentially nonsedating anticonvulsant drug. The dramatic effect of PHT and its widespread acceptance in the treatment of convulsive disorders may have tended to obscure a broader range of therapeutic uses.

A review of the literature reveals that phenytoin has been reported to be useful in a wide range of disorders. Among its reported therapeutic actions are its stabilizing effect on the nervous system, its antiarrhythmic effect on certain cardiac disorders, and its therapeutic effect on emotional disorders.

The fact that such broad therapeutic effects have been reported by many independent scientists and physicians over a long period of time would seem to indicate that the therapeutic effects of phenytoin are more than that of an anticonvulsant.

The FDA encourages the submission of formal applications, which, of course, would include the necessary supporting evidence for the consideration of approval for a wider range of therapeutic uses.

Your interest in encouraging the Department to provide a public clarification of the status of phenytoin is very welcome and I hope that this information is responsive to your concerns.

With warm regard,

Sincerely,
/s/ Elliot L. Richardson

Survey of Use of Phenytoin

There follows a survey by IMS America, Ltd. (year ending March, 1975) of the number of prescriptions of Dilantin and diagnosis and desired action.

Description of Method of Data Collection—The survey by IMS America, Ltd. is a continuing study of private medical practice in the United States; the study began in 1956. Data are obtained from a representative panel of physicians who report case history information on private patients seen over a given period of time.

Fifteen hundred physicians report four times a year on a forty-eight-hour period of their practice. Each physician fills out a case record form for every private patient treated. Case histories are returned to IMS America, Ltd. for processing. The books are coded and edited by pharmacists. All information is recorded on computer tapes, from which the monthly and quarterly reports are compiled.

Physicians in private practice are selected at random and include representatives of all specialties.

(See the following pages.)

	No. of *Prescriptions* *in*
DESIRED ACTION	*Thousands*
Anticonvulsant	3,057
Prophylaxis	255
Curb Cardiac Arrhythmia	124
Anticoagulant	121
Symptomatic	64
Pain Relief	62
Sedative-Unspecific	46
Control Heart Rate	27
Relieve Headache	24
Withdrawal Symptoms	19
Analgesic	17
Psychotherapeutic	17
Control Dizziness	17
Antineuritic	16
Reduce Tension	15
Relieve Migraine	12
Anticonvulsant and Prophylaxis	12
Sedative Night and Promote Sleep	12
Stimulant	11
Calming Effect and Tranquilizer	11
Antinauseant	10
Uterine Sedative	9
Antidepressant	7
Prophylaxis and Sedative-Unspecific	6
Antispasmodic	5
Mood Elevation	5
Antiallergic and Anticonvulsant	4
Prevent Migraine	4
Control Vertigo	4
GI Antispasmodic	4
Antihemorrhagic	3
Relieve Headache and Anticonvulsant	3
Cardiotonic	3
No Reason Given	1,820
TOTAL	5,827

DIAGNOSIS	No. of Prescriptions in Thousands
DISEASES OF CNS AND SENSORY ORGANS	2,534
Epilepsy—not otherwise specified	1,052
Grand Mal	452
Cerebral Hemorrhage	178
Cerebral Arteriosclerotic Congestion	177
Other Diseases of the Brain	176
Petit Mal	99
Trigeminal Neuralgia	89
Cerebral Embolism/Thrombosis	80
Cerebral Paralysis/Seizure	48
Stroke—not otherwise specified	38
Other Cerebral Paralysis	28
Migraine	20
Facial Paralysis	20
Late Effects of Intracranial Abscess	16
Subarachnoid Hemorrhage	10
Intracranial Spinal Abscess	10
Other Neuralgia or Neuritis	9
SYMPTOMS AND SENILITY	1,354
Convulsions	1,145
Syncope or Collapse	44
Encephalopathy	27
Jacksonian Epilepsy	26
Headache—not otherwise specified	22
Vertigo	13
Tension Headache	12
Other Ill Defined Conditions	12
MENTAL DISORDERS	656
Unspecified Alcoholism	118
Chronic Alcoholism	113
Other Drug Addiction	74
Acute Alcoholism	45
Depressive Reaction	44
Other Mental Deficiency	41
Primary Childhood Behavior Disorders	37
Other Schizophrenia	24

DIAGNOSIS	No. of Prescriptions in Thousands
Alcoholic Psychosis	23
Presenile Psychosis	21
Hysteria—not otherwise specified	21
Psychosis with Organic Brain Disorder	18
Neurotic Depressive Reaction	16
Other Pathological Personality	15
Epileptic Psychosis	13
CIRCULATORY DISORDERS	452
Disorders of Heart Rhythm	107
Myocardial Infarction	49
Arteriosclerotic Heart Disease	43
Essential Benign Hypertension	35
Other Hypertensive Arteriosclerotic Heart Disease	33
Angina Pectoris	27
Myocardial Occlusion	26
Coronary Artery Disease with Selected Complications	26
Arteriosclerosis without Gangrene	23
Myocardial Occlusions with Complications	17
Arteriosclerotic Coronary Artery Disease	17
Heart Block	9
SPECIFIC CONDITIONS WITHOUT SICKNESS	386
Surgical Aftercare	361
Medical Aftercare	25
NEOPLASMS	306
Malignant Neoplasms—Other Unspecified Sites	103
Unspecified Neoplasms Brain/Nervous System	60
Malignant Neoplasms of the Brain	41
Malignant Neoplasms of the Nervous System— Unspecified	24
Benign Neoplasms of the Brain or Other Parts of the Nervous System	22
Malignant Neoplasms of the Lung—Unspecified	19
Malignant Neoplasms of Thoracic Organs	15

(continued)

ACCIDENTS AND POISONING	228
Head Injuries	129
Other Accidents—Poisoning	35
Effects of Poisons	28
Injury of Nerves of Spinal Cord	21
Fractures	16
ALL OTHERS	212
Total[1]	6,127

[1] Since occasionally more than one diagnosis is given per prescription, the total for diagnosis is not exactly the same as the total for desired action.

When this book was published by Simon & Schuster in 1981, and Pocket Books in 1982, it contained an extensive Bibliography and Review of Phenytoin. That material has been left out of the present edition because this edition has been published to accompany *The Broad Range of Clinical Use of Phenytoin*, sent to the physicians in the United States.

If the reader does not have a copy of the Bibliography and Review we will be glad to send one on request (as long as supply lasts).

D

PRINTED BY R. R. DONNELLEY & SONS COMPANY
CRAWFORDSVILLE, INDIANA DIVISION
A QUALITY PRINTER OF BOOKS, MAGAZINES, CATALOGS,
DIRECTORIES AND OTHER PRINTED PRODUCTS